THE
PARENT'S
COMPLETE
GUIDE TO

# Ear
# Infections

# THE PARENT'S COMPLETE GUIDE TO

# Ear Infections

by
Alan R. Greene, M.D.

**≡People's Medical Society**®

*Allentown, Pennsylvania*

The People's Medical Society is a nonprofit consumer health organization dedicated to the principles of better, more responsive, and less expensive medical care. Organized in 1983, the People's Medical Society puts previously unavailable medical information into the hands of consumers so that they can make informed decisions about their own health care.

Membership in the People's Medical Society is $20 a year and includes a subscription to the *People's Medical Society Newsletter.* For information, write to the People's Medical Society, 462 Walnut Street, Allentown, PA 18102, or call 610-770-1670.

This and other People's Medical Society publications are available for quantity purchase at discount. Contact the People's Medical Society for details.

**Library of Congress Cataloging-in-Publication Data**
Greene, Alan R., 1959–
    The parent's complete guide to ear infections / by Alan R. Greene.
      p.  cm.
    Includes index.
    ISBN 1-882606-29-9 (pbk.)
    1. Otitis media in children—Popular works.  I. Title
    RF225.G74  1997
    618.92'09784—dc21                  97-8335
                                            CIP

1 2 3 4 5 6 7 8 9 0
First printing, September 1997

Cover photography: Cheryl L. Greene

*Very few people today have heroes who don't eventually disappoint. I'm fortunate that John and Gwen Greene, my parents, are heroes whose shine only increases with time. This, my first book, is dedicated to them from the depth of my soul.*

# CONTENTS

# ACKNOWLEDGMENTS

Deep thanks to Bill Adler, of Adler and Robin Books, Inc., who conceived of this book, contacted me, and offered me the opportunity to write it. He planted the seed. Thanks to my wife and parents for believing in me and to the many "HouseCalls" readers whose questions convinced me of the need for this book. They prepared the soil. No project like this can grow to fruition without the care and nurturance of many people. Thanks to Harry Verby, M.D., Patricia Soong, M.D., Karen Lee, M.D., Alger Chapman, M.D., and Jeanne Vadhanasindhu, M.D., my colleagues at A.B.C. Pediatrics, for their care and flexibility. Thanks also to the staff at A.B.C. for working with my scheduling difficulties in a cheerful way. Thanks to Garrett, Kevin, Claire, and Austin—the greatest children anywhere. Thanks to Cheryl and Christine, the other two-thirds of the "HouseCalls" team, without whom I wouldn't even be writing. What gems they are! Thanks to John and Gwen Greene, Kris Lowe, and again Cheryl for reading the manuscript and offering many needful suggestions. Thanks to Mervyn R. Blas, Kris Lowe, Pharm.D., and

Daniel Torbati for their help with antibiotic information. I am indebted as a father and as a physician to Charles Bluestone, M.D., Jerome Klein, M.D., and the other pathfinders whose work is responsible for much of our modern understanding of ear infections. Bluestone and Klein's book *Otitis Media in Infants and Children* (Saunders, 1995) is the single best reference on ear infections available today. Thanks also to Karla Morales, Charlie Inlander, Jennifer Hay, and Linda Hager at the People's Medical Society, whose skillful editing not only improved this book but also improved me. And thanks once more to my partner, Cheryl, whose love and sacrifice, particularly at this time, are gifts beyond compare.

# INTRODUCTION

# Why an Entire Book on Ear Infections?

Hoarse crying invaded my dream. As I drifted toward consciousness, I realized that my son had probably been crying in pain for several minutes. My eyes tried to focus on the clock—1:15 A.M. I stumbled into the next room and found my son in his mother's arms. "I don't know what to do," she said, handing him to me. I felt his hot tears against my cheek as I held him tight.

An ear infection is the diagnosis most likely to turn a happy, sleeping child into a crying, miserable one. This year, ear infections will send more children to the doctor than any other single cause. They will prompt more than 25 million office visits in the United States alone. More than $3.5 billion will be spent on the diagnosis and treatment of ear infections. As I held my son that night, a thought shot through my mind: Each statistic is a real child, not just a number.

I am both a physician and a father. And my son had another ear infection.

And he's not alone. The overall frequency of ear infections has been steadily increasing over the past 20 years. Antibiotics that worked so easily in years past are now less effective. These trends have combined to give birth to frustration. Whether it's the endless rounds of antibiotics, the eternity of sleepless nights, or the looming threat of surgery, children and parents around the world are sick and tired of ear infections!

One of the most exciting projects I have ever undertaken has magnetically attracted most of my free time. Economic forces are making doctors' visits briefer, less frequent, and less personal at the same time that the challenges of raising children are becoming ever more complex. This prompted my launching of "Dr. Greene's HouseCalls," an Internet Web site dedicated to using information technology to make pediatric wisdom more accessible to the public than ever before.

At http://www.drgreene.com, I receive parents' questions from all around the world. Questions flood in on an amazing variety of topics. And more questions come in on ear infections than on any other single condition.

This mom expresses the exasperation and concern shared by millions:

Dr. Greene,

My seven-month-old son was diagnosed with an ear infection three weeks ago and has been prescribed a total of four different antibiotics. In order, they are amoxicillin, Cefzil, Sulfatrim, and Lorabid. The infection has still not cleared up, and an ear, nose, and throat specialist is now suggesting tube surgery. Our regular pediatrician recommends waiting to see if things are better in the spring. What is going on here? We are totally confused! Surgery or no surgery? Or should we throw out all of the docs and start from scratch? What do you suggest? Thanks for your help!

*Jinny—A worried, sleepless, and tired mom*
*Minneapolis, Minnesota*

Jinny's confusion about what to do is common. In this book, I'll help you to sort through the conflicting advice that you're likely to hear and to chart the best course of action for your child.

Jinny is right to be concerned about the overuse of antibiotics. Ear infections are the most common reason for both short- and long-term antibiotic use in children. This is having a huge effect both on our environment and on each child who is a recipient of these antibiotics. The overall incidence of resistant bacteria is skyrocketing. The presence of resistant organisms is seven times more likely in a child who has been treated with two or three courses of antibiotics (*Contemporary Pediatrics,* March 1994). We will discuss the appropriate (and inappropriate) use of antibiotics in chapter 6.

Jinny is also right to be concerned about surgery. Chronic or repeated ear infections are more likely to place your child under a surgeon's knife than any other single cause. Tympanostomy tube insertion is the most common surgery for children. Adenoidectomy, with or without tonsillectomy, is the most common major surgery done to prevent ear infections and is also the most common major childhood surgery overall.

The only time I've ever had to experience one of my children being wheeled into an operating room was for ear surgery. As a physician, I am used to going into the operating room myself. But I disliked the empty feeling as the doors closed behind my son and I was left standing outside. He had this operation when he was only 10 months old.

Many parents dread the thought of their children having operations. On the other hand, some fed-up parents desperately want surgery for their children. In chapter 9, we'll discuss in detail when surgery is a good idea—and when it isn't!

Deep concern moved this next set of parents to take their child out of a day-care setting:

Dr. Greene,

Our son (who will soon be two years old) has been suffering from repeated ear infections. He started having problems at the age of 13 months, when he started going to a day-care facility. We understand that every time he has a cold he gets an ear infection, not to mention the possibility of allergies. Since there is no way to prevent him from getting colds in day care, we've decided to keep him at home and to take him off the antibiotics for a while to see if he gets better. If he does not get better, we may consider having tubes placed in his ears. However, we are very nervous and very concerned about the fact that he has to undergo general anesthesia for this relatively short procedure. We understand that anesthesia is required to properly complete this sensitive surgery. Can you tell us a little bit about the risks involved and whether we should be worried about this? We appreciate your advice.

*Jamal and Caterina Shamas*
*Kenner, Louisiana*

We'll examine together the huge role of day care in spreading ear infections as well as the impact of day care on the types of bacteria that cause ear infections. We'll explore the role of allergies, merely hinted at in this letter. We'll also address the issue of general anesthesia raised by Jamal and Caterina. More children are subjected to general anesthesia for the purpose of inserting ear tubes than for any other reason. We'll look together at the real magnitude of the risk.

This next question concerns hearing loss resulting from the treatment:

Dr. Greene,

My granddaughter is 13 months old and has had about one ear infection per month since she was two months old. The last bout was extremely painful for her, as she also had teeth coming in. We have heard conflicting opinions on tubes. I read your great advice on this subject. However, one opinion we got was that tubes may also cause hearing loss, thus causing a child to be a slow learner. Your opinion on this...?

*Gabrielle Ethington*
*Mesquite, Texas*

Each time a child gets an ear infection, fluid persists in the middle ear for weeks to months. Some degree of hearing loss is present whenever liquid fills the middle ear space. Since ear infections typically occur at an age when children are learning language and thinking skills, chronic or recurrent ear infections can have a profound impact on cognitive development. We'll look together at hearing loss and learning issues caused by ear infections and their treatment.

This next parent is concerned about handling the side effects of antibiotics and wonders if alternatives are available:

Dr. Greene,

My 11-month-old daughter has had an ear infection for two months. I originally took her to the doctor for a red bottom that would not heal with nystatin and Neosporin, alternately. The doctor found that her ear was a little pink inside, and we decided to put her on amoxicillin because she goes to day care and everyone there was sick. After her course of antibiotics, her bottom was not any better. In fact, it was worse! I took her back to the doctor. Her ears had gotten worse, so the doctor decided to put her on Lorabid. After three days, she was throwing up and had diarrhea. So we switched to Ceclor. Her bottom healed up, but she was getting fussier, and when she cried, she held her ears. I took her in again. Her ears weren't better, so they put her on another antibiotic, Zithromax. I knew before the 10 days were up that her ears were not better. They are now suggesting another round of antibiotics. Is this a good thing? What about the antibiotic scare that her body won't be able to fight infections and she'll become immune to antibiotics? Not to mention the yeast infections! I would like to know what to do next. Should I try some alternative medicine? I don't even know where to start. My little girl is miserable, and this is such an important time for development to be having ear infections. Thank you!

*M. C.*
*Wasilla, Arkansas*

We'll address the side effects of antibiotics in detail. We'll also look at alternative approaches to ear infections and how to evaluate them.

This parent of a five-year-old is ready to give up on conventional treatment with the hope that something less common might help to prevent ear infections:

Dr. Greene,

My five-year-old daughter has a weird pattern. She starts with a cold and a cough for three days, then runs a fever for two or three days, and then gets an ear infection. She has done this three times already. We would like to prevent the ear infection, but when we talk to her doctor, he tells us to wait for the ear infection before doing anything. Antibiotics are not, in our minds, the greatest thing for anyone. My girl does not react very well to that type of medication anyway. Are there any preventive measures we can take? Can we break this cycle in any way? Is there anything we can do to improve her immune system?

*Benoît Guilbert*
*Roxboro, Quebec*

As this dad points out, preventing ear infections is far better than treating them. Chapter 11 is devoted to preventive measures.

Besides all of the larger questions, I hear many practical concerns—such as this one about water in a child's ears:

Dr. Greene,

We are getting ready to go on vacation! My nine-month-old son gets a lot of ear infections. Should I keep him out of the water? Should I take any kind of medication with me to prevent swimmer's ear?

*Dana Martin*
*Bedford, Indiana*

We'll also discuss the latest information on water in the ears, swimming, and how these affect the ears.

For a diagnosis so overwhelmingly common, parents are too often left in the dark about ear infections. Unable to see what is going on in the ears of their children, parents must guess and then wait for their doctors to tell them if their children have ear infections or not.

Unfortunately, many doctors are too busy to explain what is really happening inside your child's ear. It's much easier to write a quick prescription for an antibiotic and move on to the next patient. If the infection is still there, just write a prescription for another antibiotic. Far more antibiotics are prescribed than are appropriate.

And all too often the wrong antibiotics are prescribed. Patterns of bacterial resistance are changing rapidly. So are the antibiotics. Eight of the 13 antibiotics commonly used for ear infections either are new or have significantly changed in the past two years. Prescribing habits developed in the past are no longer effective.

Ear tubes are a good solution for many children. But even the *Journal of the American Medical Association* (April 27, 1994) recognizes that almost 25 percent of tympanostomy tubes are put in for inappropriate reasons.

The information parents are given about these and other options is often piecemeal and contradictory. It is not surprising that parents are exasperated and confused as to how to proceed.

What is needed today is a caring and intelligent collaboration between parents and doctors. This book will not simply tell you what to do. It will not give you one right answer that will work for every child. But I am committed to giving you the information you need to work as a partner with your doctor. You will be equipped to make decisions as a team about how to best care for your child. This book will provide you with an up-to-date, thorough understanding of ear infections: their causes, their diagnosis, the variety of treatment options (with their pros and cons), and the most effective prevention strategies.

THE
PARENT'S
COMPLETE
GUIDE TO ~ Ear
Infections

*Terms printed in boldface can be found in the glossary, beginning on page 189. Only the first mention of the word in the text will be boldfaced.*

*We have tried to use male and female pronouns in an egalitarian manner throughout the book. Any imbalance in usage has been in the interest of readability.*

# 1

# The Normal Ear

## ➤ *What is the anatomy of the normal ear?*

The uniquely shaped outer ear is easy for all to see. Some ears stick out; some are close to the head. Each has its own distinct shape. Most 18-month-old children can point to an ear if asked. The shape of the outer ear focuses on the small hole that leads to a dark canal that is a mystery to most parents. Beyond what we know from "Q-Tip exploration" lies a space as unfamiliar as a forbidden temple hidden in a jungle.

The **ear canal** is a gently curved, skin-lined tube that travels through the bones of the skull. It dead-ends into the **eardrum**, or **tympanic membrane**. The eardrum is a thin, semitransparent (or translucent) membrane that separates the external ear canal from the middle ear space. Sound waves in the environment cause the eardrum to vibrate. The middle ear is an air-filled cave lying just beyond the eardrum. It is the structure that transmits and amplifies sound from the eardrum to the inner ear.

The middle ear is one of the few structures in the body that is the same size at birth as it is in adulthood. This cavity is a little

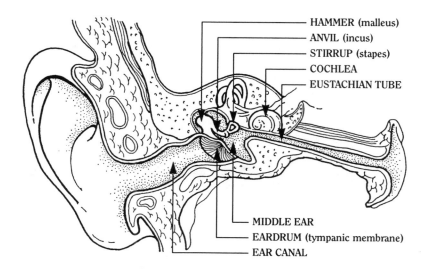

HAMMER (malleus)
ANVIL (incus)
STIRRUP (stapes)
COCHLEA
EUSTACHIAN TUBE

MIDDLE EAR
EARDRUM (tympanic membrane)
EAR CANAL

more than one-half inch tall and between one-quarter and one-eighth inch wide—a tall, narrow, air-filled box. The outer wall is the flexible eardrum; the inner wall is mucous membrane-lined bone. **Mucus** is a slippery secretion that moistens and protects the underlying tissue. It acts like flypaper, trapping any germs that make it into the middle ear.

The middle ear contains three tiny bones, or **ossicles**, that form a moving bridge across the middle ear space. The outermost of these bones is the **malleus** (or **hammer**); it attaches to the tympanic membrane. The middle ossicle is the **incus** (or **anvil**); its body has two legs, which project at right angles to one another. One of these legs is connected to the malleus, and the other is connected to the third ossicle, called the **stapes** (or **stirrup**). The stapes rests on the **oval window**, a thin membrane on the inner wall. This chain of three bones receives sound waves from the eardrum and transmits and amplifies them through the oval window to the **cochlea**, the miraculous structure that transforms sound waves into nerve signals. From the cochlea, these signals travel on to the brain.

A membrane covers all of the structures of the middle ear, including the ossicles. This glistening membrane constantly produces mucus.

## Where does all of this mucus go?

There is only one way out of the bony-walled middle ear cave. Behind the ear is a bone called the **mastoid process**. As children grow, a labyrinth of tiny, connecting caverns forms in this bone and connects to the middle ear. Mucus can enter this labyrinth. Sometimes children get **mastoiditis**, an important complication of ear infections that we'll discuss in chapter 10. The mastoid air cells, though, are a dead end. The only way for mucus to exit the middle ear system is through the **eustachian tube**.

## What is the eustachian tube?

As you will see throughout this book, the function (or dysfunction) of the eustachian tube is a critical element in ear infections. The eustachian tube is a drainage tube that goes from the middle ear to the back of the throat. The section closest to the ear is rigid; the section closest to the back of the throat is floppy.

## What does the eustachian tube do?

This tube has three important functions. For precise hearing, the most important function is ventilation or pressure equalization. In order for the eardrum to vibrate optimally in response to sound waves, the air pressure inside the middle air space must be approximately equal to the air pressure in the external canal. The eustachian tube functions as a floppy valve that allows extra air to enter or to leave relative to pressure changes in the outside air. If the middle ear were a completely sealed cavity, then rapid changes in middle ear pressure would cause the ear to burst like a balloon.

The second function of the eustachian tube is drainage of the secretions normally produced by the lining of the middle ear. The middle ear sports mucus-producing skin that is a continuation of the mucus lining of the eustachian tube, nose, and throat. Tiny hairs, or **cilia**, dot the surface of the eustachian tube. These energetic hairs move the secretions toward the back of the throat, where they are swallowed.

The third function of the eustachian tube is to protect the middle ear from bacteria, secretions, and pressure (while sneezing, for instance) from the nose and mouth. If the tube were wide open all the time, the tube would still be an effective drain, but it would not be an effective line of defense. The tube, then, typically remains closed at rest and opens only during swallowing or yawning. At these moments, the secretions drain, and the air pressure equalizes.

The proper functioning of the air-filled middle ear space allows us to hear clearly. Hearing is one of our most powerful ways of communicating with the world around us. When something occurs outside our direct line of vision, we may not be able to see the movements, but our hearing alerts us to the sounds. We become aware of events that occur at great distances and can locate sounds in space by subtle differences in the sound waves hitting our two ears. Perhaps most important, hearing opens a door to rich and varied speech, language, and music. It enables us to communicate with the people around us. Loss of hearing cuts us off from many life experiences.

Such is the importance of the tiny anatomical structures we have discussed. The smallest bones in our bodies have a big effect on our lives. And it is the unseen, unglamorous eustachian tube that is the focus of the struggle with ear infections.

# 2

# What Is an Ear Infection?

### ➤ *So what is an ear infection?*

Ear infections come in several varieties. The two main categories are **otitis media** and **otitis externa**. In medical terminology, the suffix -*itis* refers to an inflammation. *Otitis* means an inflammation of the ear. *Otitis media* means, specifically, inflammation of the middle ear. *Otitis externa* means an inflammation, or infection, of the external ear canal. Swimmer's ear is the common name for otitis externa. While both of these are common childhood problems, most people use the phrase "ear infection" to refer to otitis media, and I will follow that convention in this book. When I am speaking of otitis externa, or swimmer's ear, I will refer to it specifically.

### ➤ *Are there different types of ear infections?*

Other than the distinction between otitis media and otitis externa, otitis media is divided into two important subtypes that behave very differently. **Otitis media with effusion (OME)** is the name given to inflammation accompanied by fluid in the

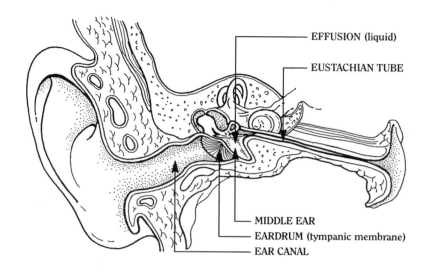

middle ear space. OME is also called **serous** or **secretory otitis media**. Children with OME act as if they feel well. Because pediatricians often discover OME at well-child examinations, OME is sometimes called **silent otitis media. Acute otitis media (AOM)** refers to fluid in the middle ear accompanied by signs or symptoms of an ear infection, such as pain, redness, or a bulging eardrum. Children with AOM act sick (especially at night) and often have fevers. After an episode of AOM, a child is often left with OME for several weeks. Care for a child with AOM is quite different from care for a child with OME.

## What is glue ear?

In some cases of OME, the fluid is thin and watery. In other cases, it is very thick. OME with a thick effusion is called **glue ear**. It used to be thought that the effusion always got thicker as time progressed. Thus, glue ear became synonymous with chronic OME. Michael Wiederhold, M.D., of the neurobiology department at the Armed Forces Radiobiology Research Institute, studied the character of ear effusions over time and found relatively poor correlation between the duration of the effusion and its thickness, or **viscosity**. The thickness had more to do with the individual ear than with time. Some ears tend to produce thick effusions, while others tend to produce thin ones (*Annals of Otology, Rhinology and Laryngology,* March/April 1980). The implications of the thickness of the fluid on hearing loss will be discussed in chapter 10.

## Are all cases of AOM the same?

Many different species of bacteria can infect the middle ear. Each of these behaves in its own way. Some are quite aggressive; some are slow and stubborn. Often a co-invasion with one or more viruses complicates the picture. The treatment most likely to be successful largely depends on which species of organism (or what combination of species) is living in a particular child's ear.

But before we get into treatment, let's take a closer look at what causes ear infections. The clearer your picture of what sets up an ear infection, the better you will be able to evaluate treatment (and prevention) options.

# 3

# What Causes Ear Infections?

## ➤ *What causes ear infections?*

As we discussed in chapter 2, otitis media is an infection in the middle ear space. Bacteria that enter the body through the ear can't get into this space to cause an infection since the path is blocked by the eardrum. Instead, bacteria enter the body through the mouth or nose. They make their way to the middle ear through the eustachian tube, that narrow channel that connects the inside of the ear to the back of the throat, just above the **soft palate**. Clearly, this tube does not exist simply to provide a secret passage for bacteria. But let's review its function, from the perspective of an itinerant colony of bacteria.

You will remember from chapter 1 that the eustachian tube is an intermittent drainage conduit to prevent the secretions normally made in the middle ear from building up and bursting the thin eardrum. Tiny hair cells in the tube propel this mucus to the back of the throat, where it is swallowed. The very thin layer of mucus that rests on the hair cells is called the **mucous blanket**.

This constantly moving blanket acts as a conveyer belt to move organisms and unwelcome particles out of the body.

When all is well, the eustachian tube remains collapsed most of the time to protect the middle ear from the many organisms that live in the nose and mouth. Only when you swallow does a tiny muscle briefly open the tube to equalize the pressure and drain the ear secretions. If any bacteria make it into the ear, they stick to the mucous blanket and are carried down the drain, helped by the little hair cells, which should flush them out.

An ear infection is the result of the eustachian tube not performing its job. If something partially blocks the tube, fluid begins to accumulate in the middle ear. Bacteria already there become trapped and begin to multiply. This is sufficient to cause an ear infection. Air in the middle ear space then escapes through the thin mucous membrane lining the middle ear into the bloodstream, producing a partial vacuum in the middle ear. This sucks more bacteria from the nose and mouth into the ear. To make matters worse, environmental irritants, including smoke and cold viruses, can kill the vulnerable hair cells. If this happens, the mucous blanket can't help to move the bacteria out. The bacteria have found a warm, protected home where they can be fruitful and multiply.

## What blocks the eustachian tube?

Respiratory infections, irritants (especially cigarette smoke), and allergies can all inflame the lining of the tube, producing swelling and increased secretions that can block the tube. These same factors can also cause enlargement of the adenoid glands near the opening of the tube, blocking flow at the outlet. Sudden increases in air pressure (during descent in an airplane or on a mountain road) can both squeeze the floppy tube closed and create a relative vacuum in the ear. Drinking while lying on the back (as babies often do when drinking from bottles) can block the slitlike tube opening. The increased mucus and saliva produced during teething can also get in the way.

## What types of bacteria cause most ear infections?

The most common cause of acute otitis media (AOM) is **Streptococcus pneumoniae** (or **pneumococcus**), which accounts for about 35 percent of cases. The next most common cause is **Haemophilus influenzae**, which accounts for about 25 percent of cases. After that comes **Moraxella catarrhalis**, which accounts for 10 to 15 percent of cases. These (*Strep pneumo, H. flu,* and *M. cat*) are the Big Three bacteria in ear infections and will repeatedly come up when we discuss treatment. The next most common species of bacteria is **group A Streptococcus**, which accounts for about 3 percent of cases. A wide variety of bacteria account for the remaining one-quarter of AOM infections.

Otitis media with effusion (OME) results from similar bacteria, although in different order. *H. flu* accounts for the largest number of cases, 15 percent, followed by *M. cat* at about 10 percent and *Strep pneumo* at about 7 percent (though this is rising rapidly). **Staphylococcus aureus** jumps into fourth place at 3 percent. The remaining two-thirds of cases of OME are caused by other organisms. These different species of bacteria vary considerably in their susceptibility to different antibiotics.

## Does getting soap or water in the ears cause ear infections?

Soap or water or bacteria that enter the ear from the outside can't get into the middle ear space to cause an infection. As we've said, bacteria enter the middle ear through the eustachian tube and cause an infection when that tube gets blocked. Although a myriad of factors can lead to a blocked tube, getting water in your baby's ears won't—so enjoy bath time with no ear worries!

### ➤ *Will keeping my child's ears clean and free of wax help to prevent ear infections?*

No, for the same reason that soap in the ears doesn't cause ear infections. For most children, there is no need to clean the wax from the ear canal. The body normally moves the wax out to the surface, where it can be wiped away with a washcloth. If the body's own mechanism isn't working, try putting a few drops of an over-the-counter earwax softener into the ear. This will make the wax thinner, so it will move to the surface more readily. If even this doesn't work, have your child's ears cleaned by your pediatrician. Inserting a cotton swab into the ear canal can cause the body to produce *more* wax and can damage the thin eardrum.

### ➤ *What about swimmer's ear? What causes it? Who gets it?*

Swimmer's ear, or otitis externa, is an infection of the skin that lines the ear canal, not of the middle ear. Bacteria normally live on the surface of this skin with no ill effect. If there is a break in the skin's normal barrier, however, the bacteria can get inside the skin and cause external otitis.

The protective barrier can be disrupted in several different ways. Prolonged wetness, the most common cause, gives rise to the name "swimmer's ear." If the ear is wet for a long time, the skin can become prunelike in the same way one's fingers and toes become soft and wrinkled when they are in water for a long time. Bacteria can easily move into the soft skin.

Others develop otitis externa from tiny scratches in the ear canal, usually from sticking a finger or some other object into the ear. This can leave the skin vulnerable to infection. The skin's barrier can even be breached when the ear becomes extraordinarily dry, causing the skin to crack. Ironically, then, swimmer's ear can be the result of spending time in desert conditions.

Swimmer's ear is more common in people who spend time in swimming pools than in people who swim in lakes. This is thought to be because the chlorine in swimming pools kills the good bacteria in the ear fairly effectively but is not as effective against the harmful bacteria hiding in the ear canal. This does not mean the water in the swimming pool is dirty. The wetness is the problem. For unknown reasons (though I suspect it might have to do with oil on the skin), swimmer's ear is not common in infants, even those whose ears get quite wet. It is particularly prevalent in preschool and school-age children.

## Do cold ears cause ear infections?

Parents from Japan to Argentina have asked me whether a child's being chilled causes ear infections. In particular, they wonder whether it's important to cover a child's ears when outside in the cold.

There is no evidence that cold ears cause ear infections. But whether breathing cold air causes ear infections is a more problematic and controversial issue.

For generations, parental wisdom has held that breathing cold air is not good for children. In particular, cold air has been thought to cause colds (thus the name). Earlier medical traditions tended to agree with folk wisdom. Over the past 15 years or so, however, the prevailing medical opinion has shifted to a different point of view. The more recent thinking is that colds, bronchitis, pneumonia, and other respiratory infections are caused not by cold air but by viruses.

I remember that when I was a pediatric resident, I was instructed to tell parents that being out in the cold made no difference—it was just an old wives' tale. I was told of scientific studies conducted at the University of Virginia in which healthy adult volunteers cavorted in the snow while wearing little clothing. They proved no more likely to catch respiratory infections than their companions indoors. Subsequently, researchers at McMurdo Station, a U.S. research base in Antarctica, conducted several important studies. (What better place to study the effect of cold temperature than Antarctica?) People in isolation at this base tended to get no colds at all—unless visitors came from the outside. Specific viruses that the visitors brought to the station worked their way through the research compound at a rather leisurely pace, approximating the rate of cold acquisition in other climates. This demonstrated that cold temperature itself does not cause colds.

The scientific studies are rather convincing, but let's consider how else cold air impacts the respiratory system. First, cold air affects mucus transport, an important defense mechanism. The entire respiratory system (including the eustachian tube and the middle ear space) is coated with a very thin mucous blanket, which traps particles and organisms to prevent them from causing infections. Proper action of this mucociliary blanket depends on the mucus having the appropriate mixture of stickiness (to catch the particles) and fluidity (to move the particles along). When this is altered by irritating chemicals, drying, cigarette smoke, or any other factor, the respiratory system becomes more susceptible to infection.

Cold air is one of these factors. It stimulates an increase in mucus production, but mucus (like other substances) becomes thicker in colder temperatures. Thus, inhaled particles are less easily cleared when a person breathes cold air—particularly through the mouth.

The second area where cold air affects respiratory health is in the nose. The hardy nose is a remarkable organ that's designed to condition inhaled air to protect the delicate internal structures.

When breathing through the nose, you may breathe in air at 40°F or 100°F, but within one-quarter of a second the air temperature is quickly brought to 98.6°. Many tiny blood vessels known as **capillaries** affect this temperature change. When a person breathes cold air, the tissue lining the nose swells as the capillaries dilate, bringing warm blood to heat the cool air. Swollen capillaries in the nose are the cause of nasal congestion (nasal congestion is backed-up blood, not increased mucus). In addition to the congestion, the mucus normally present in the nose increases and becomes thicker. Thus, cold air by itself can produce both nasal congestion and stuffiness, which again make it more difficult for the body to remove inhaled viruses and bacteria.

Piecing the available evidence together, I've reached a conclusion drawn from both traditional wisdom and current medical opinion. First, it is clear that in order to catch an infection of any type, one must be exposed to the causative organism. Second, if a person is exposed, he is more likely to get an ear infection directly—or to get a cold leading to an ear infection—if he has been breathing cold air.

As is often the case, when parents and scientists disagree, both sides tend to see important aspects of the truth. In synthesizing the two views, a more accurate view emerges.

# 4

# Who Gets
# Ear Infections
# and Why?

## Were ear infections a problem before this century?

While ear infections are more common now than ever before, they have been a common problem throughout human history. Evidence of ear infections lingers both in Egyptian mummies and in prehistoric human skeletal remains (the changes in the bone indicate a complicated course). Ear infections have pestered every society studied, but in the past the outcome was generally much worse. The stories of children in developing countries today, however, are sadly similar to those found everywhere before the advent of antibiotics.

## Why do children get more ear infections than adults?

Ear infections afflict children much more often than adults. The highest concentration of ear infections clusters in the window between six and 12 months of age. This high prevalence in early childhood has two main causes. The first is **immunologic**. Infants are born with numerous **antibodies** from their mothers that help protect them from infections. These antibodies circulate in the infants' bloodstreams in abundance for about six months, then gradually disappear. Children produce their own antibodies when they are exposed to infections and fight them off. This antibody production begins by about six months of age but generally doesn't reach significant protective levels before one year of age and often quite later. The period between six and 24 months (and particularly between six and 12 months) is the time children are most vulnerable, simply from an immunologic standpoint, both to ear infections and to colds leading to ear infections.

The other main cause is the anatomical structure of the eustachian tubes in children, which leaves them more vulnerable to infections in the ear. Although the middle air space is the same size in adults and babies, the eustachian tube in an infant averages only about three-quarter inch in length—about half as long as that of an adult. This shorter distance makes it much easier for organisms from the mouth and nose to travel up to the middle ear. Moreover, the adult eustachian tube lies in the body at an uphill angle of about 45 degrees from the horizontal, while the infant eustachian tube is either horizontal or at an angle of about 10 degrees from the horizontal. Also, the adult tube turns along its route, while the infant tube is relatively straight. This shorter, more horizontal, straighter tube affords a quick and easy trip for bacteria.

While it is easier for bacteria to make it into the middle ear of a child, it is also easier for the eustachian tube to become blocked, trapping the bacteria in the middle ear space. The location of the opening in the back of the throat is more exposed, floppier, smaller in diameter, and more apt to be blocked by secretions or by the adenoid glands, which are larger in children. Also, the tiny muscle that ordinarily opens the eustachian tube works less efficiently in infants.

An immature immune system and a more accessible eustachian tube combine to make ear infections quite a nuisance in the first years of life.

## ➤ *Are some children more prone to getting ear infections than others?*

Absolutely! Children can be divided into three groups of roughly equal size. One group gets essentially no ear infections. Another group gets sporadic ear infections (three or less in any one year and fewer than six in the first two years). The third group is prone to frequent ear infections. The definition of "prone to frequent ear infections" varies from researcher to researcher but can describe those who get at least four infections in a year or who get six ear infections in the first two years of life. These children prone to ear infections should be identified as early as possible, so they can be treated appropriately.

## ➤ *Why are some children more prone than others?*

There are several reasons. The children who are more prone might have immune systems that are not as mature and completely functioning as those of their counterparts. Their eustachian tubes might be shorter, narrower, or less efficient than average. Or there may be some reason that their eustachian tubes are more likely to become inflamed than other children's (such as allergic tendencies or exposure to environmental irritants).

## ➤ *Who is most likely to be prone to ear infections?*

Several risk factors have been identified for otitis-prone children. Ear infections, like most bacterial infections of infancy, occur more commonly in boys than in girls (for unclear reasons). Having a sibling with recurrent otitis media can make a child more likely to be prone to ear infections—though not always. (Two of my children are prone to ear infections, one has had none, and one has had a few.) Also, particularly high rates of ear infections have been observed among Eskimos and Native Americans. This seems to have a genetic basis. Ear infections run in families and genetic groups, even if the individuals change culture or location. This may have to do with inherited anatomical features or immunological weaknesses.

Children who have their first episode of otitis media before six months of age (about 25 percent of all children) are more likely to be otitis prone, as are those who are bottle-fed as opposed to breast-fed. Children in group day-care settings are also at much greater risk. If children make it to age three without ear infections, they are unlikely to ever have problems with severe or recurrent ear infections.

**Down syndrome** children and children who are born with **cleft palates** are almost universally otitis prone. So are children with a variety of uncommon craniofacial anomalies and syndromes, such as Pierre Robin syndrome, Turner's syndrome, Patau's syndrome, Treacher Collins syndrome, Goldenhar's syndrome, Apert's disease, Pyle's disease, Albers-Schönberg disease, Parrot disease, Hunter-Hurler syndrome, Mohr syndrome, and Crouzon's disease (*Otitis Media in Infants and Children,* Saunders, 1995).

## ➤ Are children with allergies more prone to ear infections?

Children with tendencies toward **eczema, asthma**, or other allergies have a higher incidence of ear infections. Allergies seem to produce inefficient functioning of the eustachian tube. This could be the result of actual inflammation and swelling of the lining of the eustachian tube or of obstruction of the outlet of the tube by the secretions in the nose.

## Does being around cigarette smoke increase the likelihood of ear infections?

Each year in the United States, secondhand cigarette smoke causes between 354,000 and 2.2 million episodes of otitis media (*Pediatrics,* April 1996). Many people think of passive smoke exposure as a minor issue. The truth is that the inhalation of secondhand smoke is a major health concern.

Exposure to secondhand smoke has now been strongly linked to a higher incidence of asthma and respiratory infections (including pneumonia) in children. Children exposed to passive smoke require hospitalization more frequently and have a greater chance of dying from sudden infant death syndrome. Girls exposed to secondhand smoke are four times more likely to get breast cancer as adults than if they are not exposed.

In August 1992, an important study appeared in *Pediatrics* that carefully examined the relationship between passive smoking and ear infections. Researchers measured the levels of cotinine (a breakdown product of nicotine) in the blood of children. By measuring blood levels of cotinine, investigators have been able to quantify the extent to which nonsmokers inhale tobacco smoke. Cotinine levels in spouses and children of smokers can even be just as high as the levels found in the smokers themselves.

The higher the concentration of cotinine in the blood in the children, the greater the frequency of acute otitis media (AOM), and the longer it took for fluid in the middle ear to clear following an acute episode. The relationship between exposure to cigarette smoke and ear infections has been clearly established.

Of course, nicotine isn't the only dangerous chemical found in the bodies of people exposed to secondhand smoke. Most of tobacco's toxic by-products reach their highest concentrations in sidestream smoke and have huge effects on nonsmokers. Still, the amount of cotinine in the blood is the best measure of how much smoke a person inhales and has made many important medical studies possible.

## How does tobacco smoke cause ear infections?

Tobacco smoke is thought to act in several ways. Smoke exposure causes increased production of mucus, which can block the eustachian tube. Also, cigarette smoke exposure damages the cilia, the hairs lining the respiratory tract, including those in the eustachian tube. This renders the normal transport function of the mucus ineffective. In addition, cigarette smoke decreases the immune system's defenses against the organisms that cause infections. Antibody-producing white blood cells are damaged. Every effort should be made to keep all children away from cigarette smoke.

## What can a parent who smokes do to help?

Thankfully, there are ways to minimize the amount of second-hand smoke children inhale. If family members smoke and are not able to stop, then restricting smoking to outside of the house certainly helps to reduce exposure.

Still, whenever you can smell the smoke, it is affecting you and your children. Masking the odor with air fresheners does nothing to help. Plenty of real fresh air is quite helpful but often impractical.

Powerful air filters are available. You can buy or rent a HEPA (high-efficiency particulate arresting) filter, which efficiently removes 99.97 percent of particles from the air. These are somewhat expensive but can save money by reducing disease (they also reduce allergy symptoms). Place HEPA filters in the rooms where people sleep. Less expensive, but also helpful, are houseplants. Plants take in the contaminated air and then release oxygen. John C. Greene, D.M.D., M.P.H., a former member of the Surgeon General's office and an expert on tobacco, has also suggested a fresh coat of paint. Tobacco residue clings to the walls and surfaces. The combination of cleaning and painting can give your home a fresh start.

Those parents reading this who do smoke can give an invaluable gift to their children by stopping. I understand that tobacco can be a real addiction and that stopping can be a monumental task. For all of us, minimizing our children's exposure to smoke is well worth the effort and expense.

## ➤ *Are children who use pacifiers more likely to get ear infections?*

In November 1995, university researchers in Finland published in *Pediatrics* their study of 845 children attending day care. They followed the children for 15 months, keeping track of behaviors that might influence the number of ear infections. These included breast-feeding, parental smoking, thumb-sucking, bottle use, and socioeconomic class.

In these children, the strongest association was with pacifier use, which increased the frequency of ear infections by 50 percent. In children younger than two years of age, pacifier use increased the average number of ear infections from 3.6 to 5.4 per year. In children between two and three years of age, pacifier use increased the number of ear infections from 1.9 to 2.7 per year. Presumably, either the sucking associated with pacifier use hinders proper eustachian tube function (which normally keeps the middle ear open and clean) or—particularly in day care—the pacifiers act as **fomites** (germ-covered objects that spread infection). The researchers suggest that pacifiers be used only during the first 10 months of life, when the need for sucking is strongest.

I believe that sucking is an important comfort measure for many babies. Moreover, children in most cultures throughout history have used some type of sucking object. In my opinion, this study suggests a take-home lesson: If your child is plagued by frequent ear infections, stopping the use of a pacifier is worth a try—certainly before repeated rounds of antibiotics or surgery.

Too often pacifier use persists into middle childhood either out of habit or because the pacifier has become the child's "security blanket"—and not out of any true sucking need. She might just as easily find comfort in something else.

### ➤ How do I get my child to stop using a pacifier?

Here are some tips that will help you wean her from pacifier use in a constructive way. First, restrict pacifier use to sleep time and stressful situations (for example, getting shots). Most children will become less attached as they experience more of the day without their pacifiers. Then make the pacifier less attractive while at the same time introducing a new comfort object. To make the pacifier less attractive, you might apply a bitter-tasting solution, such as those used to curb thumb-sucking, to the pacifier. A combination teddy bear-blanket makes a nice, comforting alternative. For an older child, you might try gathering up all of the pacifiers and taking them to the toy store for the child to trade in for the toy of her choice. For most kids, it's easier to deal with the pacifier issue before the first birthday than to wait until they become more attached and the habit becomes more ingrained.

### ➤ Do breast-fed children really get fewer ear infections? If so, why?

The rate of prolonged ear infections is five times higher in formula-fed children than in breast-fed children during the first year of life. In the second year, the rate is still more than three times higher in those who were formula-fed rather than breast-fed in their first year (*Journal of Pediatrics,* May 1995).

In a very interesting study, published in *Acta Paediatrica* in July 1982, 256 infants were divided into three categories based on their breast-feeding experience: long (breast milk was the only source of milk for six or more months), intermediate (breast-fed for two to six months), and short (breast-fed for less than two months or never breast-fed). The frequency of ear infections was lowest in the "long" group and highest in the "short" group, with the "intermediate" group falling in between. Many other studies have confirmed these findings.

What is perhaps most striking about these results is that the differences in the frequency of ear infections did not stop when nursing stopped but persisted until at least age three (which is how long the study continued).

Nursing does not guarantee that your child will be free from ear infections. You may see a formula-fed child with no ear infections, while your breast-fed child is otitis prone. Still, nursing will make the situation better for your child than it would have been otherwise.

### ➤ *Why is breast milk protective?*

A number of factors may be involved:

1. *Mechanical factors:* The facial muscles of breast-fed infants develop differently from those of their bottle-fed counterparts. This may affect eustachian tube function. Feeding position is also different in breast-fed and bottle-fed babies. During nursing, an infant almost never lies flat on her back facing straight up (unless, perhaps, Mom is a gymnast). But a bottle-fed baby frequently feeds in this position, allowing bacteria and fluid to easily travel through the eustachian tubes each time the baby swallows. It makes sense that bottle-propping (leaving a baby lying on her back with a bottle) produces a higher frequency of ear infections than other methods of bottle-feeding.

2. *Psychological factors:* Over the past decade and a half, the developing field of **psychoneuroimmunology** has repeatedly demonstrated that an individual's psychological state has a direct effect on her immune function. Perhaps the nursing experience itself directly speeds the maturation of an infant's immune system.

3. *Immunoglobulins:* All types of **immunoglobulins** (antibodies) occur in human milk. Secretory IgA, a type of immunoglobulin, attaches to the lining of the ears, nose, mouth, and throat and fights the attachment of specific infecting agents. Breast milk levels of IgA against specific viruses and bacteria increase in response to the mother's exposure to these organisms. Thus, human milk is environmentally specific milk, which the mother provides for her infant to protect against the organisms to which her infant has most likely been exposed.

4. *Attachment inhibitors:* Even breast milk from which the immunoglobulins have been removed protects against infection. This breast milk is actually able to prevent the most common ear infection-causing bacteria from attaching to mucous membranes.

5. *Lactoferrin:* Lactoferrin is an iron-binding protein that is found in human milk but isn't available in formula. It has a direct antibiotic effect on several species of bacteria.

6. *Lysosomes:* Human breast milk contains lysosomes— potent enzymes that can destroy bacteria—at a level 30 times higher than any formula. Interestingly, while other contents of breast milk vary widely between well-nourished and poorly nourished mothers, the amount of lysosomes remains constant, suggesting that they are very important.

7. *Allergic factors:* The cow's milk protein used in most formulas is a nonhuman protein. When babies are exposed to

nonhuman milk, they actually develop antibodies to the foreign protein.

While study of the connection between cow's milk allergies and ear infections is still in the beginning stages, early exposure to a foreign protein may turn out to be the primary reason formula-fed infants get more ear infections. (The effects of early exposure to foreign protein are explored in three abstracts in the January 1996 *Journal of Allergy and Clinical Immunology.*)

The mysteries of human milk have not by any means been fully deciphered. Nevertheless, it becomes clearer year after year that human milk is precisely designed for human babies. There may well be other important factors that we don't even have instruments to measure yet. Not many decades ago, immunoglobulins weren't even imagined.

Whatever the reason, breast-feeding continues to afford protection from ear infections for years after nursing has stopped.

## ➤ *Why do ear infections seem to come in waves in some children?*

The waves of ear infections parallel the peak seasons for cold viruses. This holds true even in places where winter weather is a stranger and the climate is fairly constant (for example, parts of Texas). Researchers have found that there are many more ear infections in the winter than in the summer and that those occurring in the winter take much longer to clear. Studies in both the United States and England have shown that the frequency of ear infections is at its highest between December and March and at its lowest between July and September.

Also, immediately following an ear infection, the ear is more vulnerable to another infection. It takes some time for the fluid in the ear to disappear even after the acute infection is gone. In addition, the cilia that help to protect the ear are often damaged and take time to repair. This fluid-filled middle ear with a hobbled eustachian tube is an easy target for the next bacteria that come along.

## Will my child outgrow the tendency to get ear infections?

More than 60 percent of children have experienced ear infections by the time they reach 12 months of age. Once children get past their first birthdays, the incidence of otitis declines each year—except between five and six years of age, the time most children enter school. (Children who have been in day care do not experience this kindergarten blip—they've already been exposed to most of the organisms in the community.) Ear infections after the age of seven are relatively uncommon. By this age, the skull configuration and the structure of the eustachian tube have matured dramatically, and most children have developed protective antibodies to most of the causes of ear infections.

## Why are ear infections on the rise?

Over the past 25 years, the frequency of ear infections has risen dramatically. This has taken place during the same period as the discovery of more and better antibiotics and during the same period as a significant reduction in cigarette smoke exposure. What accounts for this difference?

Some investigators point to environmental pollutants, such as carbon monoxide and airborne particulate matter, as possible causes. Others point to changes in the ozone and their effects on eustachian tube function. But the single biggest factor in the change in frequency of ear infections is probably related to the increase in day-care centers.

During their first three years in day care, children have about 25 percent more ear infections than their counterparts who are cared for at home. The rise in day-care use is sufficient to account for the rise in the number of ear infections. In 1965, only 6 percent of American preschool-age children were in group day-care settings. By 1995, this figure had risen to an estimated 50 percent—more than an eightfold increase. This number continues to rise every year. In the day-care setting, coughing and sneezing at close range are common occurrences. Respiratory viruses quite easily pass from child to child. By increasing the frequency of respiratory infections in children, the frequency of ear infections goes up as a natural result.

The rise in the number of day-care centers also affects those children who are not in day care themselves. In the same way that standing water in a community causes an increase in mosquitoes, day-care centers cause an increase in the number of **rhinoviruses** and other respiratory viruses in the communities where they exist.

## Are ear infections contagious?

Doctors frequently tell parents that ear infections are not contagious. Yet you will find that when one child gets an ear infection, not long afterward siblings and playmates often come down with ear infections as well. Why is this?

The bacteria found in one child's middle ear space are trapped and unlikely to be able to make it into another child's middle ear space. Many ear infections, however, are set in motion by a cold or another respiratory infection. These respiratory infections are highly contagious. Thus, while the ear infection is not directly contagious, the same cold that caused an ear infection in one child can spread to a second child, where it causes another ear infection.

If a child has no other concurrent infection—if the ear infection has been caused by altitude change, cigarette smoke, teething, allergies, or some other factor—then the ear infection is truly noncontagious. It would be fine for even an otitis-prone child to play with that child.

## ➤ Does flying in a plane affect a child's ears?

On a recent plane trip, a single child on the plane, who had been quite well behaved throughout the flight, screamed and moaned every moment of the 20-minute descent. We know from experience that flying affects our ears; we know intuitively that this is more difficult for children.

## ➤ What are the implications of flying with an ear infection?

I think the answer will surprise you.

Severe pain results from the stretching of the eardrum by pressure. As the plane takes off, the air inside it gets thinner. Most airlines pressurize their cabins to blunt this effect, but the pressurized cabin is equivalent to air at an altitude of about 7,000 feet. The air in the middle ear space expands along with the air in the rest of the cabin. As the air expands, it is easily forced from the eustachian tube; the eustachian tube automatically opens from the pressure. As long as there is no active, complete obstruction of the eustachian tube, the excess air exits the middle air with a popping sensation but little or no pain. Again, during ascent this process is spontaneous. A tiny muscle at the outlet of the eustachian tube automatically assists this pressure equalization.

During descent, as the air pressure rises the middle air space needs extra air to reequilibrate the pressure. However, during descent the eustachian tube does *not* spontaneously open. The tiny muscle opens the eustachian tube only during swallowing or yawning. In children, this mechanism is less efficient than in adults. Even children with healthy ears will often cry during descent. The rising pressure stretches the eardrum inward and can cause pain until air rushes into the middle air space and the ear pops.

Otitis-prone children typically have easily blocked eustachian tubes, even between ear infections. These children are more susceptible to pain when flying than their otitis-free counterparts. The next time you hear crying on descent, remember that the children are experiencing pain and that crying is another very effective mechanism for opening the eustachian tube. This is one instance where crying itself helps to solve the problem.

If the middle air space is filled with fluid, many parents and physicians are concerned about the child flying. Ironically, children generally have less pain when the ear is filled with fluid, since fluid does not expand or contract with pressure nearly as much as air does. Thus, there is minimal movement of the eardrum and no ear pain. In a study by M.H. Weiss and J.O. Frost, published in *Clinical Pediatrics* in November 1987, they observed articulate children over the age of three before a flight. The children had otitis media with effusion (OME) in one or both ears. The result was surprising at the time but in retrospect made sense: None of the children experienced pain in the ears with effusion. Those who had OME in only one ear had pain in the effusion-free ear. Children with fluid-filled ears will be safer and more comfortable when flying than their otitis-free counterparts. They do not need any particular precautions.

A child with AOM has an inflamed, tender eardrum. This reddened eardrum is particularly sensitive to stretching. Fluid is usually present in AOM and again reduces pressure on the eardrum during the flight. A child may fly with AOM, but a delay of 48 to 72 hours after initiating treatment may make the flight more comfortable.

Children who have **ear tubes**—also called **PE tubes**—may fly freely. *PE* stands for pressure equalization. As their name suggests, the tubes enable air to flow freely into and out of the middle air space without pain.

Whenever children fly, I recommend treating them with acetaminophen (Panadol, Tylenol) prior to the flight. I also recommend encouraging frequent swallowing or yawning during descent. This may be accomplished by giving the child something to drink, chewing gum, or a Life Saver-type candy.

Otitis-prone children who have at least one ear with no fluid are more likely to experience pain. I recommend treating them with topical nasal decongestant nose drops—your pharmacist can help you to choose one. Administer one or two drops of the appropriate strength in each nostril shortly before the descent begins and repeat about five minutes later if there is any discomfort. You may also want to give your child an oral decongestant prior to the flight. With this regimen, most children have safe and comfortable middle ears.

## Can a child with an ear infection receive immunizations?

Most children who have ear infections can get their immunizations without a problem. Many opportunities to protect children with immunizations have been missed due to minor illnesses. The American Academy of Pediatrics and its advisory committee on immunization practices recommend that mild illnesses, including otitis media, not delay immunizations.

In the March 6, 1996, issue of the *Journal of the American Medical Association,* researchers reported on the response to the measles-mumps-rubella vaccine among children with and without mild illness at the time of vaccination. There was no difference between the two groups, including the many who had otitis media when immunized. Unless there is a significant fever, immunizations should proceed on schedule.

# 5

# Diagnosis

*How can I know if my child has an ear infection?*

Since ear infections are the most common diagnosis in pediatrics, it is worthwhile for a parent to learn to become a Sherlock Holmes, able to notice the clues and suspect an ear infection before it becomes advanced.

First, let's dispatch a red herring. You think you've found a clue: You notice that your child, who's under age two, is pulling at his ear. What does this tell you? Careful research, published in *Pediatrics* in December 1992, found that *none* of the children studied who had ear pulling as their primary symptom actually had ear infections. Even in conjunction with other important clues, such as fever, only 15 percent of those brought in for ear pulling actually had ear infections. Most commonly, children pull their ears for other reasons: itching (caused by soap or shampoo in the ear canal or by a healing ear infection), teething, exploration, comfort, or habit. So don't jump the gun. Ear pulling is one of the most common reasons for unnecessary pediatric office visits.

## ➤ *What signs* are *helpful?*

The following signs may indicate an ear infection:

• Acute otitis media (AOM) *hurts.* As the pressure in the ear builds, the pain builds from a dull ache to a sharp, stabbing pain. The pressure dissipates intermittently, so the pain comes in waves. The pain is usually worse at night. In an older child, "My ear hurts!" is the most reliable clue. Most ear infections, however, occur in children under age two. In younger children, the best clue is evidence of pain, such as crying or screaming (usually for less than a half hour), fussiness or irritability (worse when lying down), or suddenly increased difficulty sleeping, especially at night. They may have no pain the following morning, even if the infection is still present.

• In an ear infection, fluid accumulates in the middle ear. Older children often mention a feeling of fullness or decreased hearing in the affected ear. This is difficult to detect in an infant, but you might notice shaking of the head.

• Only one-third to one-half of children with ear infections develop fevers. Temperatures over 104°F occur in less than 5 percent of ear infections. Fevers are more common in infants and toddlers than in older children. By itself, a fever is not a powerful clue, but in conjunction with the clues outlined above, it is quite incriminating indeed (the combination of true fever and pain is most often an ear infection in infants and toddlers).

• Don't let other symptoms, such as loose stools or vomiting, throw you off the trail. Ear infections are sometimes accompanied by general symptoms of illness.

• The above signs are even more suggestive if it is winter and if there is an obvious reason that the eustachian tube might be blocked—an upper respiratory infection, a change in elevation, teething, allergies, an irritant (such as cigarette smoke), or drinking a bottle while lying on the back.

Even with all of the above clues, only direct examination of the eardrum by a skilled observer can clinch the diagnosis. Conversely, it is possible for an infant to have an ear infection with no clues. Regular well-child pediatric visits are important in the first two years to screen for these silent episodes.

Let's look at two typical stories I hear in the office almost every day.

*Scenario 1:* A 10-month-old girl who had been sleeping through the night has now been waking up every night for one week. She pulls herself to a standing position in the crib and rubs her right ear. She quickly calms down when she's picked up by her parents.

This child may have an ear infection—but probably not. Most 10-month-olds regularly wake up at night. In fact, it is one of the most difficult sleep periods in life. They typically pull themselves to a standing position (they are so excited about standing at this age), and they really miss their parents (separation anxiety). They often rub their ears as a self-comforting, sleepy-time habit. Their short-term anxiety is quickly relieved when they're held. This doesn't sound like a girl who is in pain or who has an infection.

*Scenario 2:* A seven-month-old boy has had a cold for three days. Last night, he woke up screaming and remained irritable for several minutes, even when he was picked up. He felt hot to the touch. This morning, he seems completely fine.

This lad's story is the most common for an ear infection: an upper respiratory infection for several days, followed by a sudden increase in irritability, often accompanied by a fever. Because he has so much pain, being held by his parents is only partially comforting. Even though he seems better in the morning, this is a child whose eardrum should be examined. Otherwise, he will probably be feeling even worse tonight.

## Why do ear infections frequently show up at night?

There are three primary reasons that ear infections often are first noticed at night. First, the pressure in our bodies changes when we are horizontal. Thus, lying down increases congestion, ear pain, and several types of cough.

Additionally, our bodies are on 24-hour clocks called **circadian rhythms**. Hormone levels rise and fall according to this daily cycle. Some hormones help us to wake up in the morning; others help us to sleep at night. These same hormones affect how we feel pain. During the day, high levels of **cortisol**, a stress hormone, keep us from feeling some of the pain and keep our fevers in check. At night, our fevers rise, and our discomfort increases.

As if this weren't enough, our senses are barraged by stimuli throughout the day, and our brains are busy processing all of the data. At night, the amount of stimuli we are bombarded with is drastically reduced. This gives our brains an opportunity to pay more attention to the already increased level of pain.

These factors all combine to greatly amplify symptoms at night. Thus, most ear infections are noticed in the evening, after the doctor's office has closed. After a long night, the child is often happy and playful in the morning. Feeling better in the morning doesn't mean that there was no ear infection or that the infection has gone away. Ear infections often seem better each morning.

## Are ear temperatures higher in children with ear infections?

There is a correlation between a temperature taken with an ear thermometer and the probability of an ear infection. The correlation is not strong enough to make a diagnosis, but ear temperature can give another clue.

Researchers at Yale University took temperatures in both ears of children who went to the emergency room for possible ear infections. Of those who had the same temperature in both ears, only 17 percent turned out to have AOM. If the temperature in one ear was more than .5°C higher than the temperature in the other ear, 60 percent had AOM in the warmer ear (*American Journal of Emergency Medicine,* January 1995).

## ➤ *If I suspect an ear infection, do I really need to go to a medical practitioner?*

After a child has had a number of ear infections, the parents often become experts at recognizing them in their child.

As inconvenient and expensive as visits to the doctor can be, I strongly recommend—even for doctors' children—that a skilled, objective observer look in the child's ears and see each possible ear infection. This is important in order to avoid unnecessary antibiotics, to choose the best antibiotics for a particular infection, to assess the effects of long-term treatment strategies, to recognize early signs of complications, and to make wise decisions for or against surgery if that option should arise.

## ➤ *If the doctor's office is closed, should I go to the emergency room?*

On one of my rare vacations during medical school, we took a trip to Oregon. The first night there, my son Garrett woke up at about two o'clock in the morning, screaming. We tried Tylenol, rocking, lullabies—we even fed him. Nothing seemed to make him feel better. He was too young to say what was bothering him, but Dad suspected it was an ear infection.

Moved by his pain, I bundled him up, jumped in the car, and took him to a local emergency room. While we were waiting for the doctor, a thoughtful nurse gave Garrett a little pillow with pictures of tennis shoes on the cover. He clutched that tiny pillow and cuddled in close.

The doctor was eventually free from the *real* emergency, and yes, Garrett did have an ear infection. They treated his pain and started him on antibiotics. And no one scolded me for coming in.

Nor would I scold you. In fact, I would really understand. But I have since learned that there are effective ways to relieve ear pain at home (see chapter 6). Ear infections are not medical emergencies. In most cases, the extra sleep everyone gets by staying home will speed up the healing process better than a few hours' head start on antibiotics (which take days to work anyway). Besides, many managed care insurance plans no longer cover emergency room visits for ear infections.

Now that I understand ear infections better, I would not take my child to the emergency room for a presumed ear infection (though I would have his ear examined by someone else in the morning). By the time you finish this book, you will understand ear infections so well that you won't need to go to the emergency room, either.

Ten years later, though, Garrett still loves that pillow.

## ➤ Should I buy an otoscope and examine my child's ears myself?

I favor parents having as much information as possible about their children's health (or else I wouldn't be writing this book!). Still, home **otoscopes** are a mixed blessing. A bright red, bulging eardrum is difficult to miss, but many significant ear infections are much less clear-cut—even with top-of-the-line instruments. You can obtain a home otoscope from a drugstore or medical supply store for only about $30, but home otoscopes are of dramatically lower quality than the instrument your doctor uses.

This is an excellent decision to discuss with your physician, to see how it fits with his management strategy for your child. If you do decide to buy and use a home otoscope, it will still be important for your child's practitioner to have an ongoing view of your child's eardrums. The home otoscope may, however, buy you some leeway on the timing and frequency of office visits.

If I were not a physician, I'm the kind of parent who would probably buy a home otoscope. Still, although I know some parents who love their home otoscopes, most feel that they would have done just as well without.

### If I do buy a home otoscope, how can I learn to distinguish between a normal ear and an infected ear?

Most home otoscopes come with a few pictures that can give you a general idea of what to look for. An angry red, opaque eardrum bulging with fluid is probably infected; a pearly gray, translucent one is probably not. In practice, however, examining an ear is not that simple.

The best strategy is to learn to use your otoscope in conjunction with regular doctor visits. Look in your child's ears just before the doctor does and describe what you see. Then ask the doctor to describe your child's eardrums to you. Look again, and try to cement the appearance in your memory. You will learn a little more each time whether there is an infection present.

You will be at a disadvantage compared with your physician since the optics and the lighting of physician otoscopes are far superior (and also far more expensive!). In addition, the home otoscope, unlike the professional model, features no way to assess eardrum mobility, often a critical part of an ear exam. Even with much practice, some kinds of ear infections will be impossible to see, including many of those that might lead to ear tube surgery. In particular, it is dangerous to rely on home otoscopes in lieu of follow-up ear checks. The common condition of prolonged clear fluid, which can reduce hearing, is almost impossible to detect with a home otoscope—what you don't see can hurt your child. Still, you can expect to eventually become fairly proficient at identifying when your child's eardrums are acutely infected.

### ➤ When a doctor is looking in a child's ear with an otoscope, what is he looking for?

When properly positioned, the light from an otoscope shines directly on the eardrum, the end of the external ear canal. The doctor evaluates the eardrum itself for both color and translucency. Next, he evaluates the status of the middle ear, which lies just beyond the eardrum, by assessing the eardrum's position and mobility and by direct examination of the middle ear through the semitransparent eardrum, if possible.

### ➤ Does a red eardrum mean that my child has an ear infection?

Although the eardrum is typically reddened in AOM, most children with red eardrums do not have true AOM. The blood vessels of the eardrum can quickly dilate for a number of reasons, giving a red appearance. A red eardrum may be the result of a child's crying, sneezing, or fever. Again, a red eardrum by itself does not mean an ear infection. Unfortunately, many, many children unnecessarily receive antibiotics for red eardrums.

### ➤ What color is the eardrum?

The normal eardrum is the color of smoked glass or a very lightly tinted car window. Fluid never belongs in the middle ear space; it usually heralds an ear infection. A yellow color often indicates fluid in the middle ear, as seen through the translucent eardrum. Likewise, clear fluid in the middle ear may cause the eardrum to take on a distinctive blue color. A red eardrum may indicate an ear infection, but not necessarily (as discussed in the previous question). Sometimes, the eardrum appears two-toned. In this instance, one is actually looking through a translucent eardrum and seeing an air-fluid level, where there is fluid on the bottom and air on the top.

## How can I tell if the eardrum is translucent?

You should be able to look through a normal eardrum and see the classic landmarks of the middle ear. These include several parts of the malleus, the joint between the incus and the stapes, and the **round window niche**. Frequently, the **chorda tympani** nerve is also visible. Failure to see these landmarks clearly suggests that the eardrum is functionally opaque. This could be the result of an eardrum thickened by disease, or the presence of opaque fluid in the middle ear, or both. Either way, an opaque eardrum is bad.

## How is the position of the eardrum assessed?

The eardrum is normally in a neutral position, stretching across the ear canal. The short arm of the malleus is visible, but not prominent, through the eardrum. A mildly concave, or retracted, eardrum (due to a partial vacuum in the middle ear) makes the short arm of the malleus quite prominent, and what is normally the long arm of the malleus appears shortened. Severe retraction of the eardrum results in a very prominent short arm of the malleus and a severely shortened long arm. A severely retracted eardrum may actually touch the inside wall of the middle ear.

A retracted eardrum demonstrates that the eustachian tube is not functioning properly, at the very least. When even air can't get through, then bacteria-filled fluid can't, either. If there are any organisms in the middle ear, they are probably trapped.

On the opposite end of the spectrum, fullness of the middle ear space is apparent when the upper part of the eardrum becomes stretched. This obscures the short arm of the malleus.

Fullness of the middle ear can result from increased air pressure, or fluid, or both. A bulging eardrum obscures the malleus. This occurs when fluid fills the entire middle ear.

## How is the mobility of the eardrum assessed?

This is accomplished by squeezing a little rubber bulb. The process is known as **pneumatic otoscopy**. The doctor attaches a small rubber bulb to the side of the otoscope. When the otoscope is in the child's ear canal, the doctor lightly squeezes the bulb, applying positive pressure, while watching to see if the eardrum moves. Then the doctor lets go of the bulb, applying negative pressure, and again watches to see if the eardrum moves. The normal eardrum moves slightly inward with positive pressure and slightly outward with negative pressure. Decreased mobility of the eardrum means that the middle ear contains fluid or air under fixed pressure (i.e., the eustachian tube is blocked).

As you can see, diagnosing an ear infection with an otoscope is a complex task. Sometimes evaluation of the color, translucency, and position of the eardrum—as well as the appearance of the middle ear landmarks, if visible—is enough to clinch a diagnosis. If any question remains, the next step with an otoscope is to assess the eardrum mobility. With this complete set of otoscopic observations, an accurate diagnosis of an ear infection can be made most of the time.

## Do doctors ever make mistakes?

Everyone—even a trained professional—makes mistakes. Some ear infections, with red eardrums bulging with pus, are difficult to miss, even with an untrained eye. Most ear infections, however, are much more subtle than that.

It takes looking into many hundreds of ears to learn to identify ear infections reliably. In recent years, the techniques used to teach physicians to diagnose ear infections have improved. Now, a medical student's observation is typically verified—often by using an otoscope with two viewing lenses—by a more experienced observer who can see (and comment on) exactly what the student is seeing. In general, AOM is appropriately diagnosed.

Otitis media with effusion is more difficult to diagnose with an otoscope alone. The ear canal is small, dark, and easily obscured by excess wax, by sneezing, or by a squirming, crying, or feverish child. Thus, even in the best hands an accurate diagnosis of some types of ear infections is not always possible.

The general pediatrician and the ear, nose, and throat (**ENT**) specialist look in many, many more ears than even other physicians. When a child is admitted to the hospital by a different type of physician—even a pediatric subspecialist—it's not uncommon for a general pediatrician or an ENT to be asked to take a look in the ears.

### What other instruments can help to confirm the diagnosis of an ear infection?

When the situation remains murky even after pneumatic otoscopy, there are three other tests a physician might commonly order to help to pin down the diagnosis. The first is called **tympanometry**. A soft rubber probe that seals the canal is placed in the external ear. The seal must be airtight. This probe, which is attached to a tympanometer, then transmits a sound to the eardrum and middle ear. A certain amount of the sound reflects back into the ear canal. The tympanometer measures the reflected sound. This is quickly repeated as the machine changes the pressure in the ear canal, altering the stiffness of the eardrum. An eardrum that has the same air pressure on both sides—in other words, a normal eardrum—will conduct the most sound waves through it to the middle ear. A fluid-filled middle ear will decrease the transmission of sound waves and increase the amount of sound reflected back to the machine.

The results of this test suggest the amount and thickness of fluid present.

A similar machine called the **acoustic otoscope**, or **reflectometer**, does much the same thing. This handheld machine looks much like an otoscope. When it is positioned in the ear, the device emits a single sound, which then bounces back to the machine. The character of the reflected sound wave is displayed on the back of the device. The result can suggest the presence of a middle ear effusion. The advantages of the acoustic otoscope over the tympanometer are that it does not require a seal on the child's ear and that it is handheld and portable, thus requiring less cooperation from the child. Its accuracy is comparable to that of tympanometry.

Neither of these tools should be used on all children. While they are both very sensitive in picking up middle ear effusions, they also produce a large number of **false-positive** results. If they were used on a widespread basis, many children would be diagnosed with ear infections who did not, in fact, have them. These tools are most useful in situations where pneumatic otoscopy by a skilled observer still leaves questions. Their power in confirming or denying an ear infection in that situation is considerable.

The third type of instrumentation that may play a role is an **audiometer** or some other type of formal hearing test. The type of hearing test varies depending on the age of the child involved. When there is concern about the possibility of long-term middle ear effusion, a hearing test is quite important since the most significant complication we are trying to prevent is hearing loss. A normal hearing test does not rule out an infection, but it does suggest that an infection is not causing the child significant problems. On the other hand, an abnormal hearing test does not guarantee the presence of an infection, but in the presence of a suspicious ear examination, the possibility is quite strong.

A child might also be referred to an ENT, who might ॥ **otomicroscope** to get improved visualization of the eardrum and the space behind it. The otomicroscope is a powerful microscope with a lens that fits into the ear.

## How does a doctor know which bacteria are causing a particular ear infection?

Knowing the exact cause of an ear infection is of tremendous benefit. A doctor can get some clues by examining the ear. A bright red, bulging eardrum is most likely to be *Streptococcus pneumoniae*. An eardrum with blisters might result from **Mycoplasma**, an uncommon cause of ear infections. Using the patient's story, the appearance of the ear, and the latest statistics on the ever-changing local microbiological environment, the doctor must make a very educated guess.

The choice of antibiotics used is based on this educated guess. The response to the antibiotics will either confirm that guess or give powerful clues about the actual bacteria. If the child is sick enough that precise determination of the organism is essential, a process called **tympanocentesis**, or **needle aspiration**, will give accurate results. A small needle pierces the eardrum, the fluid behind the eardrum is extracted, and the organisms are then identified under a microscope or by **culture**. This procedure is *very* effective in determining the most appropriate antibiotic choice, but it is painful and invasive. It is generally performed only in children who are seriously ill or who have had a poor response to multiple courses of antibiotic therapy.

## What about cultures from the nose?

Since organisms make their way into the middle ear space through the nose or mouth, some have reasoned that using a swab from this area—a process called a **nasal swab**—would be much less traumatic than putting a needle into the eardrum and could still lead to an exact diagnosis. In studies in which tympanocentesis and nasal swabs were performed in the same children, it turned out that the organism in the ear causing the infection was almost always present in the nose or throat—but so were many other organisms. The test was **sensitive** (it contained the offending organism) but not **specific** (there was no way to tell which organism from the nose was causing the ear infection).

A negative result also has predictive value: Any species of bacteria *not* found in a nasal culture will also be absent from the ear 95 percent of the time (*Pediatric Infectious Disease Journal,* April 1996).

Unfortunately, the correlation between organisms found in the nose or throat and organisms in the middle ear has not been good enough to be clinically useful.

## How about blood tests?

Blood tests are generally not useful in the diagnosis of ear infections. White blood counts, on average, are slightly elevated with ear infections, but the individual results vary too widely to be of any real use. Each of the different organisms does produce a different average white blood cell count, but the range of counts is broad enough that they overlap considerably. Again, the information provided is not very useful for distinguishing among the different bacteria.

The organisms from an ear infection usually do not show up in a blood culture. Another blood test, called the **sedimentation rate** (or **sed rate**), evaluates the stickiness of blood cells by measuring the rate at which they settle to the bottom of a test tube. The sed rate increases slightly in children with otitis media, and again the average is different for different organisms, but there is such overlap that the test really is not clinically useful.

## ➤ *Are there any new diagnostic tools on the horizon?*

**Fluorescence emission spectrophotometry** is a thrilling new development that may dramatically change the diagnosis and treatment of ear infections. This is a painless, noninvasive way to determine which species of bacteria is causing an ear infection.

This exciting advance is being developed in a collaborative effort between the Department of Otolaryngology at Vanderbilt Medical Center and the Department of Physics at Vanderbilt University (*Laryngoscope,* March 1994). I spoke with the lead researcher, Jay Werkhaven, M.D., associate professor of surgical sciences, whose enthusiasm about the technology is contagious.

The device shines light into the ear, and the optical fluorescence through the eardrum is able to distinguish among the four most common species of bacteria that cause ear infections. The current device is too cumbersome and not available for clinical use, but a faster, handheld, fiber-optic model is already feasible. This innovation (or something like it) is likely to be a major advance in the next several years.

# 6

# Initial Treatment

## *What is the proper treatment for an ear infection?*

The proper treatment for an ear infection varies considerably depending on the location of the infection (otitis media versus otitis externa); the type of infection (acute otitis media versus otitis media with effusion); and whether this is a new infection or a recurrent one. A child's history of antibiotic use, the time interval since the last ear infection, and any other medical conditions present also influence the treatment.

There is no single best answer to this question for all children, but there are best alternatives for each of the various situations. Not all ear infections require antibiotics. For some ear infections, however, antibiotics are the best treatment available.

## *What is the proper treatment for otitis externa, or swimmer's ear?*

The symptoms of swimmer's ear are itching and/or pain in the ear. A small amount of clear discharge often accompanies the other symptoms. The ear is particularly sensitive to the earlobe being moved up and down. If a child does develop swimmer's ear, the infection can often be treated with a few drops of white vinegar placed in both ears. Put the vinegar in one ear and leave it in for about five minutes, then have the child turn her head to allow the vinegar to drain. Repeat this twice a day for three days. If the symptoms worsen or persist for more than three days, prescription antibiotic drops may be necessary. A child with diabetes should see a physician at the first signs of swimmer's ear since it can rapidly develop into a serious infection. Early, aggressive treatment can prevent this **malignant otitis externa**.

Chronic swimmer's ear is usually associated with a scalp rash called **seborrhea**. Controlling the seborrhea will often break the cycle and can be accomplished with regular use of a dandruff shampoo containing selenium (Selsun), zinc pyrithione (Head & Shoulders, Danex, Zincon), or sulfur/salicylic acid (Vanseb, Sebulex).

Swimming is generally not associated with otitis media, the other type of ear infection.

### ➤ How is acute otitis media (AOM) treated?

Many children with AOM will get better with no treatment at all. Many will not. Who gets better spontaneously and who doesn't depends primarily on the contents of the fluid trapped in their middle ears.

When needle aspiration has been used to investigate the contents of middle ear fluid, it turns out that as many as one-third of children have no bacteria in their ears (presumably they have **self-limited viral infections**—viruses that clear up with no treatment). In addition, about half of those infected with *Haemophilus influenzae* or *Moraxella catarrhalis* recover whether or not the correct antibiotic is given. In other words, about two-thirds of children recover with no treatment at all.

The remaining one-third of children, consisting primarily of those infected with *Streptococcus pneumoniae,* need antibiotics in order to recover without complications. Wouldn't it be wonderful to know in advance which children required treatment and which did not?

At the Third International Symposium on Recent Advances in Acute Otitis Media, held in 1983, participants in a panel discussion declared, "There may be some merit in withholding antibiotic therapy in selected patients who have AOM, but the criteria for identifying patients for whom this type of management will be safe have not been defined." These criteria still have not been defined.

At present, most experts feel that all children with AOM should receive a course of antibiotics. This has been proven to reduce both the rate of complications and the time before children begin to get better. I understand these recommendations and can support those who feel this way.

I am personally uncomfortable, however, with our giving antibiotics to millions of children who do not need them. The cost is immense: direct financial costs, diarrhea, allergic reactions, yeast infections, other side effects, inconvenience, battles of will, and breeding ever more resistant strains of bacteria. I eagerly look forward to the day when noninvasive optical diagnosis (or some other technique) allows us to distinguish those cases in which antibiotics are truly needed.

I will not treat a child with antibiotics if the only physical finding is a red eardrum. Until better diagnostic tools are available, I am also willing to withhold antibiotics for some children with true AOM if I am assured of another chance to look into their ears. If at the initial examination the infection does not look severe, and if the child is not otherwise at high risk (speech delay, cleft palate, history of difficulty clearing ear infections, and so on), I am willing to try refraining from treating her with antibiotics and reexamining her within 48 hours to see if the infection is resolving or getting worse. If there is clear improvement, I will skip the antibiotics and see the child later for a regularly scheduled ear recheck. If the ears are the same or worse, I will initiate antibiotic therapy.

Most doctors do not spontaneously offer this option when they diagnose ear infections. It would be appropriate to ask your doctor after any ear infection diagnosis whether you might safely wait for 48 hours, treat the child's pain, and then reevaluate the need for antibiotics. This approach can take more time in the short run but can dispense with antibiotic side effects and decrease the development of bacterial resistance.

If I am concerned based on the initial exam, the child's history, or the inconvenience of a follow-up visit, I will begin a course of antibiotics right away.

### ➤ Are there any other benefits to delaying therapy?

Children may get better faster if antibiotics are started later. Investigators at the University of Minnesota gave chinchillas ear infections. (Poor chinchillas!) The chinchillas then received either early treatment (12 hours after inoculation) or late treatment (24 hours after inoculation). Those who were treated later healed faster (*Antimicrobial Agents Annual,* August 1995).

When antibiotics kill bacteria, fragments of the bacterial cell wall can worsen inflammation. Letting the body begin fighting the infection first, before calling in the antibiotic reinforcements, seems to lessen the amount of inflammation and complications. These interesting results are preliminary. No similar studies of humans have been reported.

## If antibiotics are used, how quickly should there be a response?

A child who is getting appropriate antibiotic therapy should show significant improvement in her symptoms within 48 to 72 hours. Fluid can be expected to persist for weeks, but the child should feel and act better quickly. If the child is getting worse at any point after the first dose of antibiotics or is unimproved at 72 hours, the parent should contact the physician to reevaluate the situation.

## What can be done to ease the pain in the meantime?

While the antibiotic will take many hours to begin making the child feel better, several supportive measures can help the child to feel better in minutes or even seconds. These supportive measures include oral pain relief medications, analgesic eardrops, and local heat.

The main oral pain relief medicines are acetaminophen (Panadol, Tylenol) and ibuprofen (Advil, Motrin). Acetaminophen helps to bring down the fever and pain by acting in the brain to lower the thermostat and raise the pain threshold. It lasts for about four hours. Ibuprofen lowers the fever and reduces the pain and redness by acting at the site of inflammation. It lasts for six to eight hours. The combination of acetaminophen and ibuprofen is more powerful than either alone. The two medicines work differently: the acetaminophen in the brain, and the ibuprofen at the site of the infection. To reach maximum effect, alternate the two by first giving ibuprofen, then three hours later acetaminophen, then three hours later ibuprofen. Thus, the child always has the effect of both medicines, and one of them is always at its peak concentration. This is usually necessary for 12 hours or so and should never be necessary for longer than

48 to 72 hours. If it is, a physician should reevaluate the child.

Also available are topical eardrops that contain a local anesthetic similar to novocaine. A few drops placed in the ear canal can instantly deaden the pain and provide dramatic relief. These are available by prescription only. Parents who have otitis-prone children would do well to ask their physicians for a bottle of eardrops to have at home. The drops can help a child awakened by ear pain to get back to sleep until appropriate therapy begins the following morning. If you ever do use the eardrops, it is *very* important to have your child's ears examined the following day, even if she seems entirely better. Otherwise, a brewing, serious ear infection could be missed. These eardrops should not be used if there is fluid draining from the ear.

The most natural option for pain relief is applying local heat. Gentle heat can be applied as necessary for pain—up to 20 minutes at a time, as often as every hour. This can be done in a variety of ways, including ear cups, a warm water bottle, or warm mineral oil. Gently heat the mineral oil by holding the bottle in your hands or by setting it in a bowl of warm water. The oil should be warm (about body temperature), not hot. Then put a few drops in the ear. Some children seem to respond better to a cold pack on their ears than to heat. See which feels better to your child.

Again, none of these measures should be required for longer than 48 to 72 hours.

## How long should antibiotic treatment for AOM last?

The standard therapy for AOM is 10 days of treatment for all children. Shorter or longer regimens may be better for some infections. But since most of the research studies have been done with 10-day courses, more is known about this length of therapy than any other.

Emerging bacterial resistance has prompted research into new treatment strategies. In an article appearing in *Pediatrics* (October 1995), Jack Paradise, M.D., of the University of Pittsburgh School of Medicine, suggests new guidelines for this age of bacterial resistance. His ideas are an excellent attempt to define the new, wiser middle ground of antibiotic use. He recommends considering five factors when deciding on therapy: the child's age (older children recover more easily than younger), the season of the year (summertime infections clear most easily), the severity of the episode (mild infections rarely cause real problems), the child's history of ear infections (the fewer episodes of AOM, the more easily each one is likely to clear), and the initial response to antibiotics for the infection (prompt improvement is a good sign). If, on balance, these five factors point to a mild course, Paradise recommends limiting treatment to only five days. He further suggests that if the problem of bacterial resistance continues to escalate, it might even be possible in some of these cases to withhold antibiotics and follow the child with frequent ear examinations.

## ➤ *Why are some bacteria resistant to antibiotics?*

Whenever antibiotics are used, the most sensitive bacteria die, and the most resistant live to reproduce over time. Very resistant strains of bacteria are bred.

When antibiotics were first discovered, they had such an immediate positive effect that their widespread use proceeded almost without thought. A prescription for antibiotics, however, cannot remain the knee-jerk response to an ear infection. On the other hand, antibiotic use in ear infections cannot be abandoned. Reports from Germany in 1994 indicated the return of mastoiditis and other serious bacterial infections as the result of a lack of antibiotic treatment, or insufficient antibiotic treatment, of ear infections. We do not want to return to the preantibiotic era. Instead, we need a wise, thoughtful, new approach.

Drug-resistant bacteria pose a very real problem. *Strepto-coccus pneumoniae,* or pneumococcus, is the most common cause of AOM. There are more than 80 known strains of *Strep pneumo.* These strains vary in their responses to antibiotics. Individual bacteria within the strains also vary, much like humans vary in their abilities.

Over the past several years, resistant strains of pneumo-coccus have been emerging and spreading rapidly in the United States. Unheard of only a few years ago, these strains are showing greater resistance to more and more antibiotics each month. Even resistance to ceftriaxone (Rocephin), the powerful, injectable antibiotic, has been reported. Only one antibiotic—vancomycin (Vancocin), an intravenous medication for life-threatening situa-tions—still is completely effective against all strains. If antibiotic use continues at the current pace, I believe that it is only a mat-ter of time until resistance to vancomycin also develops.

Resistant strains are more common in children who have re-cently been treated with **broad-spectrum antibiotics**—drugs that are effective against a wide range of bacterial species. They are also more common in children in group day-care settings. Resistant strains develop in response to antibiotic use, and un-fortunately, these strains are the ones that survive the best and spread the fastest wherever antibiotics are used most. A report on the Rockefeller University Workshop, published in the *New England Journal of Medicine* on April 28, 1994, points to the massive quantities of antibiotics used in fisheries, animal hus-bandry, and other areas of agriculture as a major cause of the emergence of multiple-antibiotic-resistant bacteria.

We in medicine, however, must take responsibility for the problem. Antibiotics are commonly used to treat colds and respi-ratory viruses. More than 50 percent of children who go to doc-tors with colds get antibiotics. This unhealthy practice is even more common among affluent families (*Journal of Pediatrics*, June 1996). This must be stopped.

The most common bacterial infections in humans treated with antibiotics are ear infections. Our current situation demands that we reevaluate what has been the standard medical approach to ear infections. The need for change is clear. The best approach for the future is still coming into focus.

Antibiotics are wonderful, lifesaving tools. During the first half of the twentieth century, we keenly felt their lack as we helplessly watched bacterial infections rage. During the past 50 years, we erred in their overuse. As we enter the twenty-first century, we are beginning to appreciate the importance of balance in all that we do. Antibiotics are not necessary in the treatment of all ear infections.

## Which antibiotics are used to treat ear infections?

There are more than a dozen oral antibiotics used in the United States that have been shown to be effective in treating ear infections. These include:

- amoxicillin (Amoxil)
- amoxicillin-clavulanate (Augmentin)
- azithromycin (Zithromax)
- cefaclor (Ceclor)
- cefixime (Suprax)
- cefpodoxime proxetil (Vantin)
- cefprozil (Cefzil)
- ceftibuten (Cedax)
- cefuroxime axetil (Ceftin)
- clarithromycin (Biaxin)

- clindamycin (Cleocin)
- erythromycin-sulfisoxazole (Pediazole)
- loracarbef (Lorabid)
- trimethoprim-sulfamethoxazole (Septra, Bactrim, Sulfatrim)

Each of these has strengths and weaknesses, as I will discuss below.

### ➤ Is there a shot used to treat ear infections?

Some have advocated a single injection of ceftriaxone (Rocephin) to treat ear infections. One dose of this is about as effective as 30 doses of amoxicillin. Because this is one of our most potent antibiotics, and because bacteria inexorably develop resistance to frequently used antibiotics, I would recommend using this shot only when necessary. This would include using it for children who are very ill, who can't keep oral medications down, or who have stubborn AOM. I would then recommend giving two or three doses to completely eradicate the infection, so that no partially resistant bacteria survive to breed ever more resistant bacteria.

### ➤ What is the best antibiotic to use for AOM?

The antibiotic should be one with good results against each of the three major bacteria that cause ear infections: *Streptococcus pneumoniae, Haemophilus influenzae,* and *Moraxella catarrhalis.* The best antibiotic to choose depends on a variety of factors, including effectiveness, taste (very important to children—and parents!), side effects, convenience, and cost.

In most locations, the current first-line choice remains amoxicillin. For children who have not received many antibiotics, amoxicillin is effective, safe, inexpensive, and well tolerated. Local hospitals and health departments keep current information on local patterns of antibiotic resistance. In regions where amoxicillin-resistant *H. flu* or *M. cat* or particularly penicillin-resistant *Strep pneumo* is common, or for children who have one of these resistant strains, the first-line choice may be different. It might be amoxicillin-clavulanate, azithromycin, or a cephalosporin or a sulfa-containing antibiotic. I will discuss these other antibiotics in later sections. Amoxicillin has been the first-line choice for many years, but it is unlikely to remain the first-line choice much longer, as bacteria become more resistant and as other antibiotics offer more convenient dosing schedules. In fact, in many areas people are already choosing one of the other drugs as a first-line choice.

### Is it important that my child take all of the antibiotic?

The most common reason for antibiotic failure is lack of getting the complete course—either skipping doses or stopping prematurely. This usually occurs because of taste, side effects, or inconvenient dosing regimens. If the antibiotic requires refrigeration but is kept at room temperature, the doses given will be ineffective. Make sure you and your doctor pick an antibiotic that will work for your family.

Partial courses of antibiotics, aside from being less effective, also contribute to the problem of emerging bacterial resistance. The most susceptible bacteria die in the first few days. The hardiest survive longer and, if the course is stopped prematurely, go on to expand their population in the nose of your child. This can make your child's next infection more difficult to treat and is dangerous for all of us.

### What side effects should I watch out for?

Side effects include:

• *Allergic reactions:* These can occur with any antibiotic. They most commonly appear as hives or skin rashes. If your child develops hives or skin rashes while on antibiotics, call the doctor promptly. Rare, serious allergic reactions can cause breathing difficulties, shock, or even death.

• *Diarrhea and other gastrointestinal symptoms:* When antibiotics kill the disease-producing bacteria in the ear, they also sometimes kill the beneficial bacteria in the intestines. Thus, all antibiotics can produce gastrointestinal symptoms, such as diarrhea and abdominal pain.

• *Yeast infections:* Antibiotics' ability to destroy beneficial bacteria can also lead to yeast infections. Yeast is common in our environment and can thrive on skin depleted of beneficial bacteria, particularly if the skin is inflamed—as the buttocks often are from diarrhea. Giving live-culture yogurt or acidophilus milk to children on antibiotics may help to reduce yeast infections and gastrointestinal side effects by replacing the beneficial bacteria in the gut. Frequent diaper changes and air-drying are helpful. An over-the-counter antifungal cream (such as Lotrimin) can be helpful if a diaper rash begins to appear.

Other side effects are specific to individual antibiotics and will be discussed below.

## ➤ Which antibiotics taste the best?

Nonparents sometimes scoff at the importance of taste. But anyone with children knows that the taste of an antibiotic makes a big difference, both in the amount of an antibiotic that a child actually ingests and in the amount of work that goes into treating an ear infection.

From time to time, reports of blind taste tests of antibiotics appear in the medical literature, with different antibiotics topping the lists. Many manufacturers claim that theirs taste best. Most manufacturers do their best to make the medicines taste good to children, but this is less possible with some compounds than with others.

Cefaclor (Ceclor), cefprozil (Cefzil), loracarbef (Lorabid), cefixime (Suprax), and amoxicillin routinely get high marks for taste. Many kids turn up their noses at cefuroxime axetil (Ceftin), cefpodoxime proxetil (Vantin), and clarithromycin (Biaxin)— even the new, clearly improved flavor.

I used to have a T-shirt that read *"De gustabus, non disputandum est"*—or "It's silly to argue about tastes." My own kids don't like Ceclor (a perennial favorite) but enjoy Biaxin. Go figure!

---

### RANKING OF 12 ANTIBIOTICS USED FOR EAR INFECTIONS BY TASTE TEST

1. loracarbef (Lorabid)
2. cephalexin (Keflex)
3. cefixime (Suprax)
4. cefaclor (Ceclor)
5. cefprozil (Cefzil)
6. amoxicillin-clavulanate (Augmentin)
7. penicillin V (V-cillin K)
8. penicillin V (Veetids)
9. cefpodoxime proxetil (Vantin)
10. trimethoprim-sulfamethoxazole (Sulfatrim)
11. erythromycin-sulfisoxazole (Pediazole)
12. dicloxacillin (Dynapen)

Source: *Pediatric Infectious Disease Journal,* February 1994

## ➤ *Are generics just as good as name brands?*

The Food and Drug Administration requires that the generic have the same active ingredient(s), strength, and dosage form as the brand-name equivalent. The generic must have the same efficacy and safety. But the flavors and inactive ingredients may vary.

Recently, researchers in Long Island, New York, conducted a randomized, double-blind taste test of generic versus brand-name antibiotics. Their study pitted Pediazole against generic erythromycin-sulfisoxazole and Bactrim against generic trimethoprim-sulfamethoxazole. They found that children three to 14 years of age took the preparations equally well but preferred the taste of Bactrim over the generic trimethoprim-sulfamethoxazole (*Pediatric Infectious Disease Journal,* January 1996).

To me, currently available generic cefaclor tastes identical to Ceclor. Again, it doesn't matter what other children prefer. It comes down to what your child will take.

## ➤ *Which antibiotics are given only twice a day? Or better yet, once a day?*

Not too long ago (in the 1970s), the most commonly used antibiotic for ear infections, ampicillin, needed to be given four times a day. This required a noontime dose, often at day care or school. When amoxicillin, amoxicillin-clavulanate (Augmentin), and cefaclor became available at only three times a day, it was a major convenience. Three-time-a-day dosing, however, still requires a midafternoon dose. Even if day care and school aren't problems, it's still difficult for an adult to remember to take a medicine three times a day for 10 days, much less to give it to a child— particularly if battles develop over taste.

Thankfully, amoxicillin-clavulanate and cefaclor have recently been made available with convenient twice-a-day dosing. Other preparations, such as cefuroxime axetil, cefprozil, clarithromycin, loracarbef, and trimethoprim-sulfamethoxazole, also offer the convenience of morning and evening administration.

Even more convenient are once-a-day preparations, such as cefixime (Suprax), cefpodoxime proxetil (Vantin), and ceftibuten (Cedax). Azithromycin (Zithromax) is the most convenient of all, with a standard course of only once a day for five days.

### ➤ *Which antibiotics don't need to be refrigerated?*

Azithromycin, cefixime, cefuroxime axetil, clarithromycin, clindamycin (Cleocin), loracarbef, and trimethoprim-sulfamethoxazole do not require refrigeration. This is particularly convenient when traveling. For older children, both chewable tablets and those that are swallowed afford this convenience.

### ➤ *Which antibiotics are available as chewable tablets?*

Amoxicillin and amoxicillin-clavulanate come as chewable tablets. The new amoxicillin-clavulanate chewable tablets, which became available in July 1996, taste better than ever before but, to me, are still not as good tasting as amoxicillin chewables.

### ➤ *Which antibiotics are the best deal financially?*

Sometimes parents are shocked to go to the drugstore to pick up a prescription, only to find a staggering price tag of $100 or more. Most antibiotics cost less but can still be quite expensive. The amount of antibiotic needed depends on a child's weight, so sometimes the cost varies among children.

Some antibiotics, including amoxicillin, trimethoprim-sulfamethoxazole, and erythromycin-sulfisoxazole, are available in generic form and are *considerably* less expensive than antibiotics that are not available as generics. If they work, they are clearly a great deal.

The newer antibiotics tend to be the most expensive at four

or five times the cost of generics, unless like azithromycin—with five doses instead of amoxicillin's 30—they are expensive per dose but reasonable per course of therapy.

### ➤ Can antibiotics be given with food?

This depends on the particular antibiotic. Penicillin, ampicillin (not often used for ear infections anymore), ceftibuten, loracarbef, and the solid form of azithromycin are not well absorbed when there is food in the stomach. They should be taken one hour before or two hours after a meal. Otherwise, their efficacy is significantly decreased.

Amoxicillin-clavulanate and clarithromycin have fewer gastrointestinal side effects if taken when there is already food in the stomach.

Any of the antibiotics except ceftibuten and loracarbef may be mixed with a small amount of formula, milk, fruit juice, or food, if it makes administration easier.

### ➤ Can antibiotics be given with other medicines?

Antibiotics can interact with other medicines. Make sure your doctor and pharmacist know what other medications your child is taking. See below for information pertaining to individual antibiotics.

### ➤ Which oral antibiotics are safe for children younger than six months?

Clindamycin may be used at any age but is reserved for serious infections. Amoxicillin, amoxicillin-clavulanate, cefaclor (ages one month and older), erythromycin-sulfisoxazole (ages two months and older), trimethoprim-sulfamethoxazole (ages two months and older) and cefuroxime axetil (ages three months and older) are the only ear infection antibiotics approved for children in the first six months of life.

### How do the antibiotics most often used for ear infections compare with each other?

See the chart.

| Drug | Dosing Schedule | Flavor of Liquid | Liquid Needs Refrigeration | Chewables | Generic | Appropriate First-Line Therapy |
|---|---|---|---|---|---|---|
| amoxicillin | 3 times daily for 10 days | Bubble gum | Yes | Yes | Yes | Yes |
| amoxicillin-clavulanate (Augmentin) | 2 times daily for 10 days | Orange-raspberry | Yes | Yes | No | Alternative |
| azithromycin (Zithromax) | 1 time daily for 5 days | Banana, cherry | No | No | No | Alternative |
| cefaclor (Ceclor) | 2 times daily for 10 days | Strawberry | Yes | No | Yes | Alternative |
| cefixime (Suprax) | 1 time daily for 10 days | Strawberry | No | No | No | No |
| cefpodoxime proxetil (Vantin) | 1 time daily for 10 days | Lemon creme | Yes | No | No | No |
| cefprozil (Cefzil) | 2 times daily for 10 days | Bubble gum | Yes | No | No | Alternative |
| ceftibuten (Cedax) | 1 time daily for 10 days | Cherry | Yes | No | No | No |

*chart continued on next page*

*chart continued from previous page*

| Drug | Dosing Schedule | Flavor of Liquid | Liquid Needs Refrigeration | Chewables | Generic | Appropriate First-Line Therapy |
|---|---|---|---|---|---|---|
| cefuroxime axetil (Ceftin) | 2 times daily for 10 days | Tutti-frutti | No | No | No | No |
| clarithromycin (Biaxin) | 2 times daily for 10 days | Fruit punch | No | No | No | Alternative |
| clindamycin (Cleocin) | 3 or 4 times daily for 10 days | Flavored for pediatric use | No | No | No | No |
| erythromycin-sulfisoxazole (Pediazole) | 3 or 4 times daily for 10 days | Strawberry-banana | Yes | No | Yes | Alternative |
| loracarbef (Lorabid) | 2 times daily for 10 days | Strawberry bubble gum | No | No | No | Alternative |
| trimethoprim-sulfamethoxazole (Septra, Sulfatrim, Bactrim) | 2 times daily for 10 days | Cherry | No | No | Yes | Alternative |

## ➤ *What do I need to know about amoxicillin?*

Since it was first introduced in the 1970s, amoxicillin has remained the first-line antibiotic choice in the treatment of AOM. This is beginning to change as resistant strains are emerging in some areas, but amoxicillin is still the first choice in most areas. Amoxicillin is usually not a good choice, however, to treat persistent, prolonged, or frequent ear infections. It has a failure rate of almost 60 percent in these situations. Theoretically, amoxicillin is a good choice as a **maintenance antibiotic** (an antibiotic given over a long period of time to prevent ear infections), but each bottle of the liquid remains active for only 10 to 14 days, necessitating many trips to the drugstore for long-term use.

Amoxicillin comes in a pleasant-tasting bubble gum-flavored liquid ("the pink stuff"), chewable tablets, or capsules to swallow. The liquid form must be kept refrigerated to remain active; it should be shaken well before each dose. Amoxicillin must be administered three times a day. It may be taken without regard to meals and may be mixed with food or juice if your child prefers to take it that way. Generic amoxicillin is commonly used and is a good, economical choice.

Amoxicillin should not be given to children who have known allergies to any penicillin or who have infectious mononucleosis. It should be used cautiously in children with kidney damage since it is supposed to exit the body through the kidneys. It should not be given with the drug allopurinol, a medicine for gout. Allopurinol is rarely prescribed for children, but if a breast-feeding mother is taking this medicine, amoxicillin is probably not the best choice of antibiotic for her child.

The most common side effects of amoxicillin are diarrhea, yeast infection, allergic reaction, and a nonallergic rash usually seen five to nine days into the course of the drug. (A rash does not necessarily mean that the child should stop taking the drug, but it should be reported to the physician.) Nausea and vomiting are uncommon side effects. Rare side effects include **colitis** (inflammation of the colon), anemia, low white blood cells, low platelets, inflammation of the kidneys, and shock. It is one of the best-tolerated antibiotics.

## ➤ *Why doesn't amoxicillin always work?*

When it was first introduced, it was truly a wonderful choice since it was very effective against the Big Three ear infection-causing bacteria (*Streptococcus pneumoniae, Haemophilus influenzae,* and *Moraxella catarrhalis*). Amoxicillin, like all members of the penicillin family, is called a beta-lactam antibiotic because of its molecular structure. It works by destroying the cell wall of bacteria but not of mammalian cells.

Over time, many of the *H. flu* and most of the *M. cat* have learned to make an enzyme called beta-lactamase that destroys beta-lactam antibiotics like amoxicillin. In 1970, all 108 strains of *M. cat* were susceptible to amoxicillin; by 1980, only 85 percent were susceptible; and by 1990, only 25 percent were susceptible. Currently, about 70 percent of strains of *H. flu* isolated from children's ears remain susceptible. Thankfully, many other antibiotics are available for these resistant bacteria.

More frightening, however, is the recent emergence of resistant strains of *Strep pneumo*. When penicillins were first introduced more than 40 years ago, all strains of *Strep pneumo* were dramatically sensitive to all penicillins. In 1977, multiple-drug-resistant strains of *Strep pneumo* were reported in South Africa. Over the past 20 years, these have spread throughout the world, with their highest incidence in Spain, France, eastern Europe, and now parts of the United States. These may soon cause the obsolescence of amoxicillin for otitis media and are a blazing challenge to abandon the indiscriminate use of antibiotics in favor of a more selective, balanced approach.

## ➤ *What do I need to know about amoxicillin-clavulanate (Augmentin)?*

When bacteria began producing the enzyme beta-lactamase to destroy beta-lactam antibiotics like amoxicillin, scientists created a new antibiotic called Augmentin. It contains amoxicillin and clavulanate, a potent inhibitor of the bacteria-produced beta-lactamase.

When amoxicillin-clavulanate was introduced in 1984, it restored the full original potency of amoxicillin. What's more, this efficacy has so far remained undiminished over the years. The problem was, amoxicillin-clavulanate had more side effects than amoxicillin.

Partly because the antibiotic is more effective (and thus destroys more of the beneficial bacteria in the intestines) and partly because of the clavulanate, Augmentin produced more yeast infections and more gastrointestinal problems—especially diarrhea and cramping—than amoxicillin.

Over time, the formulation and dosage have been adjusted, reducing the frequency, the total dose, and the amount of clavulanate. The most recent version, released in July 1996, seems to be quite well tolerated and is available in convenient twice-a-day dosing.

Amoxicillin-clavulanate comes in a pleasant-tasting orange-raspberry-flavored liquid, chewable tablets (which taste better than previous versions but are still nothing to look forward to), and film-coated tablets to swallow. The liquid should be shaken well before each dose and must be kept in the refrigerator. It should be discarded after 10 days. The medicine can be mixed with formula, milk, fruit juice, soft drinks, or food. There are fewer side effects if there is already something in the stomach when the medicine arrives.

Other side effects, drug interactions, and precautions are the same as for amoxicillin. Augmentin is not available as a generic.

Amoxicillin-clavulanate is an appropriate choice either as a first-line agent (for a brand-new ear infection) or when other antibiotics have not worked. It remains effective against any of the common ear infection bacteria. In fact, Augmentin is often the standard with which other antibiotics are compared.

## What do I need to know about azithromycin (Zithromax)?

New on the scene in 1996 (approved for use in children), azithromycin boasts convenient once-a-day dosing for only five days. Azithromycin remains in the body, making a five-day course the equivalent of a 10-day course of other antibiotics.

Azithromycin belongs to the macrolide family of antibiotics, along with erythromycin, erythromycin-sulfisoxazole (Pediazole), and clarithromycin (Biaxin). These antibiotics are unaffected by beta-lactamase-producing bacteria. They work by damaging the bacteria's apparatus for producing proteins. Without making proteins, bacteria can't grow or reproduce, and they soon die.

Azithromycin is quite effective against the Big Three bacteria as well as a number of other ear infection-causing bacteria. It is weakest against *Haemophilus influenzae*. So if it doesn't work, the next antibiotic selected should be effective against *H. flu.*

Azithromycin comes in banana- and cherry-flavored liquids, which taste pretty good, and in capsules. The capsules are most effective when taken on an empty stomach either one hour before or two hours after a meal. Azithromycin should not be taken concurrently with an aluminum- or a magnesium-containing antacid.

Care should be taken when administering azithromycin to a child who's also on theophylline, digoxin, or seizure medication, as the blood levels of these medicines could be affected. Also, since the drug is eliminated from the body by the liver, care should be used in children with liver damage.

Azithromycin is quite well tolerated, with only 5 percent of children experiencing diarrhea, 3 percent experiencing nausea, and 3 percent experiencing abdominal pain. All other side effects occur in less than 1 percent of children. Jaundice and rare allergic reactions are the most serious side effects reported.

If a child has had nausea, vomiting, diarrhea, or abdominal pain with erythromycin, azithromycin is still an appropriate choice and will probably produce fewer side effects. If, however, a child has had an allergic reaction to erythromycin, with hives or breathing difficulties, an antibiotic from a different family should be selected, if possible.

Azithromycin is considered an alternative first-line choice for ear infections. It is first line in children allergic to penicillins, cephalosporins, or sulfa drugs or in settings where ease of use is a major issue. Azithromycin is also a good choice if there is a treatment failure after 48 to 72 hours of another drug.

Zithromax is not available as a generic.

### ➤ *What do I need to know about cefaclor (Ceclor)?*

Cefaclor is a member of the cephalosporin family and a cousin to the penicillins. Like penicillins, it works by disrupting the bacterial cell wall. Unlike penicillins, it is not a beta-lactam molecule and thus is not as easily thwarted by beta-lactamase-producing bacteria.

Cefaclor is a broad-spectrum antibiotic. It works against many ear infection-producing bacteria, including the Big Three. When it was introduced, it was the Cadillac of ear infection medicines because it worked great, tasted great, and carried a hefty price tag.

For amoxicillin-resistant bacteria, cefaclor was an ideal choice because it worked so well and was much easier to take than early regimens of amoxicillin-clavulanate. In fact, it has been so successful and has enjoyed such widespread use that bacteria are now beginning to figure out ways to resist it. Treatment failures are becoming a little more common each year. Cefaclor is still effective, but its star is not burning as brightly as it once did.

Cefaclor is a reasonable choice as a first-line agent but is no longer recommended for persistent otitis, with treatment failures approaching 40 percent in 1995. As a broad-spectrum drug, it does not make a good choice for a maintenance antibiotic to prevent ear infections.

Cefaclor comes in a delicious strawberry-flavored liquid or in capsules to swallow. The liquid is given twice a day; the capsules, three times a day. The liquid must be refrigerated and should be discarded after 14 days.

Cefaclor, like any cephalosporin, should not be given to anyone with a severe allergy to any penicillin since the two drug families are closely related structurally. It may be given to children in whom amoxicillin causes rashes. Cefaclor exits the body via the kidneys and should be used with caution in cases of kidney failure. People should not ingest alcohol in any form—even cold medicine elixirs—within 72 hours following a cefaclor dose.

The most common side effects are allergic reactions (showing up as rashes) and gastrointestinal problems. About 2.5 percent of people taking cefaclor will develop a gastrointestinal problem such as diarrhea. Because cefaclor is a broad-spectrum antibiotic, it can cause colitis by destroying many beneficial as well as harmful bacteria. Cefaclor can also cause a serum sickness-like reaction: rash, swelling, arthritis, and fever. Thankfully, this reaction resolves by itself after the antibiotic is stopped. A host of other side effects have been reported, but overall, cefaclor is well tolerated. It has been proven to be safe for children as young as one month of age.

In 1996, a generic cefaclor became available. It is an identical product in every way to the name brand.

## ➤ *What do I need to know about cefixime (Suprax)?*

Cefixime became popular for three reasons: It was the first ear infection antibiotic to feature once-a-day dosing; it has a crowd-pleasing strawberry taste; and the liquid does not need to be refrigerated.

Cefixime, like cefaclor, is a cephalosporin. It is less effective against *Streptococcus pneumoniae* (the number one cause of ear infections) than any of the other antibiotics discussed thus far but is quite effective against *Haemophilus influenzae, Moraxella catarrhalis,* and many of the less frequent organisms. This makes cefixime an outstanding choice following a treatment failure by a drug active against *Strep pneumo* but not a great choice as a first-line agent.

It is also quite effective against gastrointestinal organisms, and as such, this broad-spectrum antibiotic can cause gastro-intestinal side effects in about 30 percent of children. The great majority who stop taking cefixime because of side effects do so because of gastrointestinal problems.

As with all cephalosporins, cefixime should not be used following a serious allergic reaction to a penicillin or another cephalosporin (except perhaps the cefaclor serum sickness-like reaction). Cefixime may even be used in kidney failure. Its safety has not been demonstrated for children under six months old.

Besides the strawberry liquid, cefixime is available as a film-coated tablet. There is no generic.

## ➤ What do I need to know about cefpodoxime proxetil (Vantin)?

Cefpodoxime proxetil is a very strong, extended-spectrum cephalosporin, effective against even more bacteria than most broad-spectrum antibiotics. It is very stable in the presence of beta-lactamase and thus can be effective when penicillins or even other cephalosporins fail. Its pattern of efficacy is most similar to amoxicillin-clavulanate or cefuroxime axetil.

Because of its extended spectrum, cefpodoxime proxetil can have increased gastrointestinal side effects, with diarrhea occurring in 17.8 percent of infants and toddlers. Sometimes these side effects are quite severe.

Cefpodoxime proxetil comes in film-coated tablets and in a lemon-creme liquid. The aftertaste is even worse than the first swallow. The manufacturer didn't try to make cefpodoxime proxetil taste bad; this is a powerful compound with a powerful taste. The manufacturer actually did a good job of disguising it. Some kids even like cefpodoxime proxetil. It helps the taste if the cefpodoxime proxetil is cold and is mixed with something strong, like chocolate syrup, or with chilled fruit juice. Quickly rinsing the mouth or "chasing" the medicine with some raspberry jam will make the next dose easier to get in. The pill form is about the size of a Tic-Tac. Hidden in some pudding or applesauce, it often goes down easier than the liquid. Cefpodoxime proxetil is given only once a day.

Cefpodoxime proxetil offers excellent results against stubborn, persistent otitis, including those cases caused by many of the resistant *Strep pneumo*. This strong drug is not necessary for most ear infections, but I'm very glad it's available. There is no generic form.

## ➤ *What do I need to know about cefprozil (Cefzil)?*

Cefprozil is a popular, pleasant-tasting cephalosporin that works very well against most ear infection-causing bacteria except beta-lactamase-producing strains—against which it still works moderately well. It is particularly good against *Strep pneumo,* the most common cause of ear infections. It is comparable to cefaclor, before resistance to Ceclor began to emerge.

Cefprozil should not be given to someone with a known serious allergic reaction to a penicillin or a cephalosporin. It should be used with caution in someone with kidney failure. It has been shown to be safe in children as young as six months.

Only 2 percent of children discontinue cefprozil due to side effects. The most common side effects are nausea (3.5 percent), diarrhea (2.9 percent), and diaper rash (1.5 percent).

Cefprozil comes in film-coated tablets and in a bubble gum-flavored liquid. The liquid must be kept refrigerated and should be discarded after 14 days. It is given twice a day. There is no generic.

## ➤ *What do I need to know about ceftibuten (Cedax)?*

Ceftibuten was new on the market in 1996 and was very heavily promoted to physicians. It is the newest of the oral cephalosporins and is most similar to cefixime (Suprax). Ceftibuten features once-a-day dosing and a popular cherry taste. The big advantage compared with cefixime is a lower incidence of diarrhea (4 percent), the major side effect of both drugs. It has been shown to be safe in children as young as six months.

Ceftibuten is very effective at killing both *Haemophilus influenzae* and *Moraxella catarrhalis,* but it is somewhat less effective against *Strep pneumo* (the most common cause of ear infections). Because of this, ceftibuten is not a good choice as a first-line agent. It is a reasonable choice as a follow-up, if the first antibiotic was particularly strong against *Strep pneumo* but less strong against *H. flu* or *M. cat.*

Ceftibuten should be taken on an empty stomach at least one hour before a meal or two hours after a meal. It is best not to mix it with food or juice, although this would usually not be necessary. If your child has diabetes, note that the liquid contains one gram of sugar per teaspoon. The liquid lasts for 14 days if kept refrigerated. There is no generic available.

## What do I need to know about cefuroxime axetil (Ceftin)?

Cefuroxime axetil is another broad-spectrum cephalosporin trying to pick up a piece of the huge market created by cefaclor. The liquid form was introduced in 1995 and has great broad-spectrum efficacy. Like amoxicillin-clavulanate (Augmentin), it works well against every one of the top eight causes of ear infections, including many of the resistant *Strep pneumo*. It is too broad spectrum and too expensive to use as a first-line agent, but it can be quite useful after a treatment failure or in combined infections involving an infection of the skin or pneumonia.

Cefuroxime axetil comes in a tutti-frutti flavor that has not been at all popular with the children in my practice. It is given twice a day. Otherwise, it is well tolerated, causing diarrhea in only 3.7 percent of children and nausea or vomiting in 3 percent of children. It may be taken with or without food but should not be taken with any type of antacid.

Cefuroxime axetil comes in film-coated tablets and in liquid. The liquid does not need to be refrigerated but should be discarded after 10 days. The same allergy precautions apply as with other cephalosporins. Cefuroxime has been shown to be safe in children as young as three months old. There is no generic form.

## ➤ *What do I need to know about clarithromycin (Biaxin)?*

Clarithromycin is one of the macrolide antibiotics, along with azithromycin (Zithromax) and erythromycin-sulfisoxazole (Pediazole). This family of antibiotics is a good first choice when there is a cephalosporin allergy or a significant penicillin allergy.

The first edition of clarithromycin had a poorly accepted taste. The current formulation, which arrived in 1996, tastes better. Unlike other antibiotics, the liquid contains microencapsulated granules, which give it a gritty sensation. Clarithromycin should not be refrigerated. It should be thoroughly shaken before administration, and the mouth should be thoroughly rinsed afterward to prevent a horrid aftertaste if the granules remain and the coating melts. Often children like the medicine better if it is mixed with orange juice or chocolate syrup.

The medicine is given twice a day for 10 days. It may be given with or without food. There are potential drug interactions with many other medicines, including asthma medicines, seizure medicines, and some antihistamines. It is very important that your doctor and pharmacist know all other medications that your child is currently taking.

Clarithromycin works quite well against *Strep pneumo*—even some of the resistant strains—and against *M. cat.* Its strength against *H. flu,* while better than the earlier macrolides, is still not great. Still, clarithromycin is a very effective second-line antibiotic.

The most common side effects in children are vomiting (6 percent), diarrhea (6 percent), and abdominal pain (3 percent). There is no generic available.

## ➤ What do I need to know about clindamycin (Cleocin)?

Clindamycin is a third-line antibiotic: It should be used only when AOM persists after appropriate first- and second-line choices have both failed. Clindamycin is superb against infections caused by penicillin-resistant *Strep pneumo*. The major drawback is that this powerful drug can cause serious colitis and/or diarrhea. The intravenous form is known to occasionally cause fatal diarrhea. While the oral form is not nearly as dangerous, notify your doctor immediately if any diarrhea occurs while taking clindamycin.

Clindamycin is given three or four times daily for 10 days. It may be given with or without food. It is available in tablet and liquid forms. The liquid form should not be refrigerated. It is flavored for pediatric use—but most children find it unpalatable. There is no generic available.

## ➤ What do I need to know about erythromycin-sulfisoxazole (Pediazole)?

Pediazole is a combination of a macrolide (erythromycin) and a sulfa (or sulfur-containing) drug (sulfisoxazole). It has been around for many years. It is considered a reasonable first-line choice for children with penicillin and cephalosporin allergies. It must be kept in the refrigerator.

Although erythromycin-sulfisoxazole is effective against some strains of *Strep pneumo, H. flu,* and *M. cat,* it currently is less effective against each of them than azithromycin and clarithromycin. Moreover, the gastrointestinal side effects are considerably more common: Five times as many children stop taking erythromycin-sulfisoxazole because of side effects. Combine that with a strawberry-banana taste that ranked 11th out of 12 antibiotics in a major study, a three- or four-times-a-day dosing schedule, and the longest interval before an improvement in symptoms of any ear infection antibiotic, and it makes one wonder why physicians would ever prescribe it.

Compared with other macrolide antibiotics, such as azithromycin and clarithromycin, the main advantage of erythromycin-sulfisoxazole is cost. The generic form is very inexpensive. Even though erythromycin-sulfisoxazole is less effective than other choices, it still does work most of the time. Even though many children experience side effects, a great many don't. And even though many antibiotics taste better, most kids don't object to the taste. Many families who do not have insurance coverage for prescriptions would rather try a generic medicine first and then use a more expensive preparation only if there is little or no improvement. Cost-conscious insurance companies often urge this same course of action.

## What do I need to know about loracarbef (Lorabid)?

Loracarbef is a new antibiotic brought out by the manufacturers of Ceclor. Structurally, it is almost identical to cefaclor, but it is more effective (at least in the test tube) against *H. flu* and *M. cat* and just as effective against *Strep pneumo*. Loracarbef also has fewer side effects. Notably, cefaclor's serum sickness-like reaction has not been reported. Diarrhea is the most common side effect at 6 percent. Safety and efficacy have been demonstrated in children as young as six months of age.

Loracarbef comes in a strawberry bubble gum-flavored liquid that was top-ranked in a study comparing the tastes of 12 antibiotics. The liquid may be stored at room temperature. It also comes in capsules for older children and adults. Loracarbef is given twice a day either one hour before or two hours after eating. No generic is available.

## ➤ *What do I need to know about trimethoprim-sulfamethoxazole (Septra, Sulfatrim, Bactrim)?*

Septra, Sulfatrim, and Bactrim are all brand names for a combination antibiotic called trimethoprim-sulfamethoxazole. This antibiotic is in widespread use.

Trimethoprim and sulfamethoxazole are both compounds that block the internal production of folic acid, or folate. The combination product, trimethoprim-sulfamethoxazole, is far more effective than either ingredient alone.

We all need folic acid, a B-complex vitamin, to survive. Most bacteria must manufacture their own supplies of folic acid. Animals are able to get what they need from what they eat. Thus, trimethoprim and sulfamethoxazole are relatively safe for humans, yet lethal to many bacteria.

The sulfamethoxazole component is a sulfa drug. It causes fewer side effects than other sulfa drugs, but its side effects can still cause problems.

The most common significant side effects are allergic skin reactions. Most of these are mild, but occasionally they are quite severe. Trimethoprim-sulfamethoxazole should be discontinued at the first sign of a skin rash. Excess sun exposure should be avoided by anyone taking trimethoprim-sulfamethoxazole.

Other side effects have been reported in virtually every organ system in the body, but the other main concern is kidney problems. Sulfa drugs may crystallize in the urine. These crystals can cause bleeding, urinary obstruction, or kidney damage. This is best prevented by using the most soluble of the more than 150 different sulfa drugs—such as the sulfamethoxazole in Septra, Sulfatrim, and Bactrim—and by drinking lots of fluids while on the medication.

Trimethoprim-sulfamethoxazole should not be given to

children with folic acid deficiency. Also, it interacts with phenytoin (Dilantin), methotrexate, and anticoagulant medications, so it should be used cautiously—or not be used at all—if these other drugs are being taken. Trimethoprim-sulfamethoxazole should not be given to children under two months of age. I would also think twice before giving it to children who have severe allergies or asthma.

Trimethoprim-sulfamethoxazole is given twice a day. It may be kept at room temperature, but it must be protected from exposure to light.

Trimethoprim-sulfamethoxazole is prescribed by some doctors as an alternative to amoxicillin for first-line therapy. While it still works fairly well against *H. flu,* both *M. cat* and *Strep pneumo* are steadily becoming more resistant. Trimethoprim-sulfamethoxazole should not be used to treat persistent infections: It has the highest reported failure rate—75 percent—of all of the ear infection antibiotics. It may be a reasonable choice as a preventive antibiotic. A generic version is available.

### How effective are antibiotics in treating AOM?

More than 250 excellent research studies have tried to measure how antibiotics affect the cure rate for AOM. Overall, 90 to 95 percent of children who are treated with an appropriate first-line antibiotic are cured of AOM within 10 to 14 days (otitis media with effusion—continued fluid in the ears without symptoms— may continue longer). This is a great track record!

But remember that about two-thirds of children with AOM spontaneously get better, with or without treatment. Some experts put this figure as high as 70 to 90 percent. Thus, antibiotics improve the cure rate, but only by 5 to 30 percent (probably 10 to 15 percent, on average). In other words, if seven children with AOM were treated with antibiotics, only one of them would be cured who would not have been cured without the antibiotic. Antibiotics provide a modest boost in the number of ear infections cured (*Pediatric Clinics of North America,* December 1996).

The main reasons to treat ear infections with antibiotics are (1) to speed up symptom relief, (2) to decrease the rate of complications, and (3) to cure the children whose infections would not be cured without antibiotics. Several studies have shown that children treated with antibiotics recover much faster than children treated with a **placebo**, even when the number of children in both groups who eventually recover is almost equal. More important, children treated with antibiotics have a complication rate that's 200 times less than that of children who don't receive antibiotics for AOM. Complications of ear infections will be discussed in detail in chapter 10.

## Are there any other drugs, besides antibiotics, that can be given for ear infections?

Repeated ear infections can be so frustrating that they have prompted many people to try other treatments with the hope of improving the situation.

The two treatments that, along with antibiotics, have the most advocates in mainstream medicine are **steroid medications** and **antihistamine/decongestant combinations**. Both of these treatments are aimed at reducing blockage of the eustachian tube, which makes intuitive sense.

In light of the many different approaches to treating ear infections, the American Academy of Pediatrics, the American Academy of Family Physicians, the American Academy of Otolaryngology–Head and Neck Surgery (ear, nose, and throat doctors), and the U.S. Department of Health and Human Services' Agency for Health Care Policy and Research convened an interdisciplinary panel of experts to sift through the mountain of literature on ear infections and to provide guidelines based solidly on well-designed research studies. Their report was published in July 1994.

The panel made no comment on many of the possible treatment options because adequate research was unavailable. However, they felt that there was sufficient evidence to comment on decongestants, antihistamines and steroids.

This panel recommended against using antihistamines and decongestants, either alone or in combination. Although it would make sense that relieving congestion should help, studies that looked at the use of these medications showed no improvement in outcome over the use of antibiotics alone. With no established benefit, the side effects and cost were considered prohibitive. Individual children do differ in their sensitivities to medications, so I cannot tell you that a prescription-strength decongestant will not help your child. But I can tell you that every attempt to prove its efficacy in clinical studies has failed.

The panel also recommended against the use of steroid medications. There is limited scientific evidence that steroids might be somewhat effective in speeding up the clearance of middle ear fluid, but the adverse effects of steroids outweigh their possible benefits.

Apart from antibiotics, none of the medications carefully studied has been shown to be of benefit. Still, this is an exciting time in ear infection research, as many alternatives are just now being carefully looked at.

# 7

# Alternative Treatments

> How were ear infections treated before
> the advent of antibiotics?

Prior to the antibiotic era, many children were followed with simple observation. The otitis media would resolve on its own, either by a spontaneous perforation of the eardrum or by drainage through the eustachian tube. In the meantime, the symptoms were managed with painkillers (particularly aspirin or opium) and local applications of heat. The most common medical intervention when a sick child was taken to a physician, or perhaps a barber, was to lance the eardrum to allow the pus to drain.

You may notice that careful observation, pain control, and eardrum surgery remain important parts of therapy today.

Before antibiotics became part of the therapeutic arsenal, many children did not do well. In 1932 at Bellevue Hospital in New York City, 27 percent of all pediatric admissions were due to serious complications of otitis media (*Otitis Media in Infants and Children,* Saunders, 1995). The incidence of significant complications (which will be discussed in chapter 10) plummeted with the advent of antibiotics.

Today, otitis media in developing countries resembles the disease as it appeared before antibiotics were available.

## ➤ *What other types of therapies are used for ear infections?*

A broad range of alternative treatments is available. Approximately 11 percent of children in the United States use some type of alternative medicine (*Pediatrics,* December 1994). Homeopathy is used by a great many people and will be discussed in the next question in this chapter. Aromatherapy makes use of essential oils such as chamomile, basil, hyssop, lavender, and rose. The oil is carefully rubbed around the ear in an attempt to reduce inflammation and cure infection. Herbal therapy makes use of common herbs such as echinacea, goldenseal, mullein, peppermint, slippery elm, tansy, and willow, usually in the form of teas and gargles. Chinese herbalists use a different selection of herbs and aromatic stimulants. Hydrotherapy involves the inhalation of steam to reduce blockage of the eustachian tube and hot baths to improve circulation. Acupuncture and acupressure both have adherents who report cures of ear infections. Reflexology purports to cure ear infections by stimulating the ear reflexes on the feet. Crystal therapists select crystals to be worn to stimulate the body's own healing mechanisms. Naturopaths might recommend fasting, hydrotherapy, salt packs for the ear, or herbal remedies. Color therapists might suggest wearing deep blue colors around the head to promote healing. Spiritual healers often rely on prayer or faith to facilitate a cure. Chiropractic manipulation is thought to enhance the drainage of an infection through the eustachian tube (*The Hamlyn Encyclopedia of Complementary Health,* Hamlyn, 1996; *The Complete Book of Complementary Therapies,* People's Medical Society, 1997).

Let's look more closely at one of these therapies.

## ➤ *What is homeopathic medicine, and how are ear infections treated?*

Homeopathic medicine, like allopathic, or conventional, medicine, has a rich and controversial history. Homeopathy began in the late 1700s and early 1800s, a time when medical doctors relied primarily on bloodletting, intestinal purging, induced vomiting, and blistering of the skin to treat their patients' maladies. A brilliant physician named Samuel Hahnemann, M.D., was dissatisfied with the status quo. He was bothered both that current treatments were harsh and dangerous and that they failed to produce good results.

Hahnemann began to recommend exercise, good diet, and fresh air to his patients. He believed that healing came from God and nature and that the physician's role was only to gently encourage this natural process.

Over time, he became increasingly disturbed by the lack of evidence to support popular conventional therapies. He believed that each medicine should be tested to see what it really did before it was used as a treatment.

Hahnemann set out to prove the effects of the common remedies of his day. His first experiment was with quinine, known to treat malaria and its raging fevers. When he took quinine while well, it produced a fever. This and subsequent experiments gave rise to his Law of Similars: Remedies that produce specific symptoms in well persons are effective in treating ill persons with the same symptoms. This is where the name *homeopathy*—meaning "like the disease"—came from.

Hahnemann's treatments tended to produce an initial worsening of symptoms, often followed by a cure. To make the process more agreeable, he decided to dilute the substances he was using. The surprising result was that the remedies became even more potent. This led to the second law of homeopathy, the Law of Infinitesimals: The smaller the dose of a medicine, the more effective it is in stimulating the body to heal itself.

---

### *HOMEOPATHIC MEDICINES*

While your child's ears should be examined by a skilled expert if you suspect an ear infection, you might want to start with a home remedy, especially if the symptoms begin at night. Homeopathic remedies are labeled according to how diluted the active ingredient is. The label contains a Roman numeral and a number. An X on the label means that 1 part active ingredient was added to 9 parts distilled water to make a 1-in-10 dilution, while a C on the label means that 1 part active ingredient was added to 99 parts distilled water to make a 1-in-100 dilution. The number next to the letter indicates how many times the original dilution was carried out. Thus, for a 5X dilution, a 1-in-10 dilution was carried out five times to make a 1-in-100,000 dilution. For a 5C dilution, a 1-in-100 dilution was carried out five times to make a 1-in-10,000,000,000 dilution. If you need a 6C preparation, you can purchase a 5C dilution and dilute it again by 1 in 100 to reach a 1-in-1,000,000,000,000 dilution. At even a 5X dilution, a homeopathic remedy is unlikely to contain even a single molecule of the original active ingredient. Homeopaths say, however, that the once-present ingredient reorients the water molecules, much like a pillow retains the impression of a sleeper who has risen.

---

Over the past two centuries, the respect accorded homeopathy has varied widely. Currently, there is a resurgence in its
popularity. I greatly admire the gentleness, the reliance on the
body's own healing mechanisms, and the bent toward prevention
that are central to homeopathy.

I am quite comfortable with the idea of seeing a homeopathic
doctor as a supplement to seeing your regular physician. Conventional pediatricians are trained to recognize an amazing
array of uncommon childhood illnesses. Exciting new develop-
ments occur almost daily. Pediatricians are also trained in the
complexities of normal childhood development. We are experts in
many areas—but we are still novices in others. For ear infections, I would certainly recommend ongoing supervision by a
skilled physician.

*The Family Guide to Homeopathy* (Simon and Schuster,
1989) cautions that even with homeopathic therapy, otitis media
with effusion may take many months to clear up. For each of the
remedies described below, the appropriate dose is one drop, one
little pill, or just enough granules to cover the fingernail of your
pinkie. Appropriate treatment for otitis media with effusion
(OME) includes one of the following:

• Flint (6C potency), taken four times daily for seven days if
OME is associated with a sinus infection

• Mercurous chloride (6C potency), taken four times daily for
seven days if the child has phlegm and swollen adenoids

• Potassium chloride (6C potency), taken four times daily for
seven days if the child has a runny nose and cough

• Pulsatilla (6C potency), taken four times daily for seven days
if the blockage tends to clear outdoors

Some homeopaths also recommend a general self-help
solution for people with otitis media with effusion: lemon juice

diluted with an equal volume of saline solution. Put three drops in each nostril three times a day for five days (unless there are nosebleeds).

*The Family Guide to Homeopathy* recommends that ear pain always be promptly investigated by your doctor or homeopath. For acute otitis media (AOM), homeopathic therapy might include one of the following:

• Aconite or wolfsbane (30C potency), taken every half hour for up to 10 doses if the child is restless or the attack is brought on by a cold

• Belladonna (30C potency), taken every half hour for up to 10 doses if the child is flushed with a hot face and fever, stares, engages in excited and incoherent behavior, or has unusual sensitivity to touch

• Pulsatilla (6C potency), taken every half hour for up to 10 doses if there is pain and pressure behind the ear and the child is weepy

Homeopathy began with a desire to prove the effects of medicines by careful experimentation at a time when allopathic medicine was based simply on tradition. Today, 80 percent of allopathic treatments still have never gone through clinical trials. Thankfully, ear infection treatments buck this trend. Most have been rigorously tested, and many new trials are now ongoing.

Today, however, controlled studies of homeopathic treatments are almost nonexistent. A few studies have demonstrated the benefits of homeopathic treatments for hay fever, migraine, and diarrhea, but as yet there is no good evidence to support homeopathic treatments for ear infections. Instead, these gentle treatments are touted based on individual testimonials in much the same manner as the barbarous practices of conventional medicine two centuries ago. Many people swear that these remedies work. I hope that they're right.

The Agency for Health Care Policy and Research published important, well-founded guidelines for managing ear infections. They wanted to make recommendations regarding homeopathic treatments and sought evidence to support their recommendations. They were unable to find any reports on homeopathic treatments that contained information obtained in randomized controlled studies. As a result, they felt unable to comment on the real benefit—if any—of these remedies.

As, alas, am I.

The problem with all of the above therapies is that to date, no randomized controlled study has ever shown any of them to be more effective than a placebo.

## What's the big deal about randomized controlled studies?

If 100 children with otitis media with effusion receive chiropractic manipulation for one month and 60 of them are cured, and if the treatment is continued for two more months and 90 of them are cured, then chiropractic manipulation has done absolutely nothing. If 100 children with frequent episodes of AOM take garlic concentrate for a year and their annual rate of ear infections drops by one to three episodes, then taking garlic has done absolutely nothing (*Pediatric Clinics of North America,* December 1996).

Since so many ear infections heal on their own, it becomes very difficult to tell if a suggested remedy really works or if it is another example of the body's own healing power. While individual testimonials about certain treatments can be inspiring, they can lead us to put our trust in solutions that do not actually help. But what's the problem if the child feels better? Who cares *why* he feels better?

There are several problems. Some nonhelpful treatments (such as certain types of surgery) are both risky and expensive. Some nonhelpful treatments (such as many prescription medications) can have side effects. Some nonhelpful treatments (such as many of the alternative practices) can give false reassurances and lead to decreased expert follow-up—which can in turn lead to undetected, serious complications.

To benefit the individual child and to build our knowledge of otitis media on a firm foundation, well-designed clinical studies are very important. In a well-designed study, the definitions must be clear. For example, AOM might be defined as an inflammation of the middle ear with the presence of fluid and accompanied by specific signs and symptoms. The study might require the diagnosis to be confirmed by two or more independent observers and perhaps tympanometry and acoustic reflectometry. Microbiological diagnosis is also important: Samples of the middle ear fluid are examined to determine which bacteria or viruses are actually involved.

The children should then be randomly divided into two or more groups, so the proposed treatment can be compared with other options. These different groups must have similar characteristics—age, sex, ethnicity, and so on.

The effect of the treatment should be evaluated by unbiased individuals who do not know which treatment each child has received. These are "blind" individuals. A study is "double-blind" if even the patients don't know which treatment they have received. This can remove reporting bias (people who know they have received placebos are more likely to report more symptoms).

Ongoing evaluation using objective measurements should be carried out at about three days (to identify treatment failure), at about two weeks (to identify relapse), and at about one month (to identify recurrence).

Each time research methods like this are used, we gain another piece of the otitis media jigsaw puzzle. Each isolated testimonial only adds to the maze of options, unless subsequent careful evaluation is done.

Even if studies have not yet been done, you can try an alternative therapy if you are confident that it is safe, if the potential benefits outweigh any potential risks, and if careful follow-up is ensured. Next, I will give you an example of an unproven alternative treatment being used in a constructive, collaborative way.

## ➤ *What about ear candles?*

I first heard about ear candles from Carolyn, the mother of a delightful patient of mine. This old folk remedy is also known as ear coning, or ear cleansing. Modern practitioners trace the roots of ear candling back to Egyptian ceremonies. It is one of the techniques used to treat ear infections in the preantibiotic era. Candling is used as a traditional healing method in many cultures around the world.

Today in the United States, you might find a chiropractor, a massage therapist, or an herbalist who is skilled in ear candling. Or you might attend a workshop where you can learn to do candling yourself. The technique is simple. While the child lies on his side, a hollow candle that resembles a soda straw is gently placed in the outer edge of the ear canal. The base of the candle is surrounded by a drip guard, and a flame-retardant cloth is draped over the head of the patient. The candle is lit with a match and allowed to burn for 10 to 15 minutes while the patient is encouraged to relax with massage, music, or a pacifier. Usually, each ear is treated with two candles. The entire process is found by most to be quite relaxing. Many wander in and out of sleep during treatment.

I have heard many explanations by proponents of how ear

candling is supposed to work. Most agree that the warmth and gentle vacuum produced by the low flame soften the earwax and pull it out of the ear canal. In fact, ear candling is used by many as a comfortable way to remove excess wax. Some proponents of ear candling go on to suggest that the heat and gentle vacuum pull the infection through the eardrum and out of the body and also pull toxins from the nerves, fluid from the sinuses, and excess lymph fluid from throughout the body. Others suggest that it removes blockages to a natural acupuncture point and thus functions as an alternative to acupuncture. Some say that the heat causes a realignment of the bones of the skull. Some suggest that the ear candles even pull impurities out of the internal carotid artery. None of these explanations seems likely to me; some are completely implausible.

I believe that if ear candles have any direct effect on ear infections, it is that the warmth triggers the opening of the eustachian tube. Perhaps the warmth also increases blood flow to the area, sending white blood cells and other immune factors to the site of the infection. There has never been any scientific evidence that ear candles benefit ear infections, but it is certainly possible.

When Carolyn brought her daughter to my office with a mildly inflamed eardrum that was poorly mobile, she asked if she might try ear candling rather than antibiotics for her daughter. Since the child had no fever, her symptoms were otherwise mild, and the examination of her ear was consistent with a mild infection, we agreed that she would have ear candling performed and I would again examine her ears in 48 hours. The first time we did this, the ear infection resolved by the time she came back to the office. Whether hers was one of the two-thirds of ear infections that would otherwise have spontaneously resolved, we will never know. Still, we were able to avoid antibiotics and ensure that her ears cleared. Since then, we have followed this same procedure a number of times. Sometimes her ears clear, and other times when she comes back we start the antibiotics.

I feel that this is an ideal model for the use of an alternative therapy.

8

# Ongoing Treatment

## ➤ *What if my child doesn't get better after the initial treatment?*

Once treatment is initiated, the child with acute otitis media (AOM) should be noticeably better within 48 to 72 hours. Continued symptoms should be considered a treatment failure. Contact the treating physician to reevaluate the situation. Another antibiotic should probably be prescribed. This antibiotic should be selected to address any potential weaknesses in the first antibiotic. Particular care should be taken to cover beta-lactamase-producing bacteria by using an antibiotic such as amoxicillin-clavulanate (Augmentin), ceftibuten (Cedax), cefuroxime axetil (Ceftin), cefixime (Suprax), or cefpodoxime proxetil (Vantin) or to cover resistant *Streptococcus pneumoniae* by using an antibiotic such as amoxicillin-clavulanate, clarithromycin (Biaxin), clindamycin (Cleocin), cefuroxime axetil, cefprozil (Cefzil), cefpodoxime proxetil, or azithromycin (Zithromax). Which medication is prescribed depends on the first antibiotic used, the local bacterial resistance patterns, and the history of the individual child.

In the past two years, three antibiotics have had particularly high failure rates when used to treat **persistent acute otitis media.** Amoxicillin has failed in 57 percent of cases; cefaclor (Ceclor) in 37 percent of cases; and trimethoprim-sulfamethoxazole (Septra, Bactrim, Sulfatrim) in 75 percent of cases (*The Sanford Guide to Antimicrobial Therapy 1996,* Antimicrobial Therapy, Inc., 1996).

### What if my child gets better but starts acting sick again within a few days?

The child who experiences improvement within 48 to 72 hours but then develops symptoms again, either while still on an antibiotic or within four days of finishing an antibiotic, is said to be having a relapse. A relapse is far more likely to represent a resurgence of the original ear infection than the appearance of a new ear infection. Perhaps the original infection was caused by a mixed group of organisms, some responsive to the original antibiotic and some not. Or perhaps the bacteria were only intermittently responsive to the original antibiotic. In any event, a relapse should be treated the same way as a treatment failure.

### When is an ear infection likely to be a fresh one rather than a continuation of a previous one?

If a child's latest ear infection began at least five days after the child completed the previous antibiotic course, the infection is likely to be a new one. This is particularly true if the child is in day care or around many other kids. For a few weeks following an ear infection, a child is at increased risk for catching a new one since the defense mechanisms in the ear have not yet returned to normal. In particular, the middle ear often still contains fluid, and the little hairs (cilia) that keep washing away the bacteria and fluid are often still damaged. An infection occurring five or more days after completing an antibiotic course is called **recurrent acute otitis media**—a subsequent ear infection that is not a continuation of the first one. Investigators have studied the bacteria in recurrences by inserting a needle through the eardrum and withdrawing fluid. These studies have shown that *Strep pneumo* and *Haemophilus influenzae,* the bacteria that predominate in initial ear infections, also predominate in recurrences (*Otitis Media in Infants and Children,* Saunders, 1995). Thus, a recurrence can be treated with the same antibiotic as the first infection or with another first-line antibiotic.

If there is doubt as to whether a particular infection is a relapse or a recurrence (e.g., the ear was never examined after the original infection), it is probably wisest to treat it as a relapse— but to make sure that the antibiotic has excellent *Strep pneumo* coverage. Cefixime and ceftibuten are probably not ideal in this situation.

### ➤ *If an antibiotic worked for my child's ear infection last time, why doesn't my doctor just prescribe the same one instead of making me take my child into the office again?*

A wide variety of bacteria can cause ear infections. The type of bacteria is very important since different bacteria are sensitive to different antibiotics. Just because your child has another ear infection, there is no guarantee that the same type of bacteria is responsible. Many parents have the perception that one type of antibiotic works well for their children while others do not. Actually, the efficacy of a given antibiotic at a given time depends on the bacteria currently infecting your child. This may have changed dramatically since the last infection. Bacteria evolve very rapidly, and the last antibiotic your child was on has influenced which bacteria might be thriving in your child now.

## Why does my doctor insist on an ear recheck visit even if my child is acting better?

Even when children are acting well, they can have lingering ear infections. They can have ongoing evidence of AOM or simply have ears filled with fluid. This can result in hearing loss or other, more serious complications. Also, an ear recheck can pin down whether there is complete resolution between ear infections, thus distinguishing between relapse and recurrence. This has important implications both for immediate antibiotic choice and for long-term management.

Ear rechecks are particularly important during a child's first two years. This is the time when ear infections and their complications are most common and most troublesome. Also, these children are less verbal. They may communicate ear pain effectively but are not likely to be able to identify and communicate a sense of fullness or popping in the ear.

Children over age three who are articulate and acting well, with no symptoms, can often be safely cared for without ear rechecks.

## What is the doctor looking for at an ear recheck?

The doctor hopes to find the ear infection cured, with a normal-looking eardrum and middle ear space. Sometimes, though, the doctor sees a reddened, distorted eardrum or continued pus in the middle ear. This should be regarded as a treatment failure, and the child should receive another course of antibiotics. Sometimes the eardrum is retracted. This indicates that the eustachian tube is still blocked. I will discuss this condition in chapter 10.

More often than not, the doctor finds that the eardrum has returned to normal but that the middle ear is filled with a clear, yellow fluid. This is called an effusion. Although this fluid usually still contains bacteria, antibiotics are often not necessary in treating otitis media with effusion (OME). This fluid does affect the hearing, however. It is important to know whether this fluid is present in order to treat it properly.

## Do ear rechecks sometimes result in the overuse of antibiotics?

I believe that ear rechecks are an important part of caring for a small child with otitis media. When used properly, they can minimize antibiotic use. All episodes of AOM, though, end with an effusion for some time. The average effusion is present for 21 days. In the past, before experts became concerned about antibiotic overuse, most children with fluid still in their ears received another round of antibiotics. Since the average effusion is present for 21 days, most children got a second round, and most were better by the next ear recheck. Today, many physicians still fail to distinguish between AOM and OME and treat indiscriminately. This is one of the biggest causes of too many rounds of antibiotics.

## What can I do if my child has frequent ear infections?

That depends on the type of ear infection. In children with many ear infections, one of three possibilities applies. Some children have repeated episodes of AOM with complete clearing between attacks. Some children have chronic OME, or persistent, prolonged fluid in the middle ear. Each time they go back for an ear recheck, there is still fluid in the ear. Some children have sporadic bouts of AOM superimposed on chronic OME. These three groups of children should be cared for differently.

First, we'll discuss those who have recurrent bouts of AOM that clear between episodes. These children are the most likely to benefit from **prophylactic antibiotics**, or preventive antibiotics. We'll look at the treatment of OME, with or without superimposed bouts of AOM, later in this chapter.

## How many episodes of AOM is considered frequent?

I begin to consider further treatment options for children who have three or more episodes within a six-month period or four episodes in a year. The decision to progress to further therapy may be modified by the time of year (I'm less likely to institute new therapy in the spring), by the age of the child (I'm less likely to institute new therapy for a three-year-old than for a two-year-old), and by the recent frequency of infections. I am more likely to institute prophylactic antibiotics for a child after four or more episodes within a six-month period or six episodes in a year. Many studies have shown that prophylactic antibiotics reduce the frequency of ear infections.

## What are prophylactic antibiotics?

Prophylactic antibiotics are medicines that are given in advance in order to prevent ear infections. They are also called maintenance antibiotics. The use of prophylactic antibiotics can reduce the frequency of ear infections by 40 to 90 percent. This strategy is most effective in children under the age of two. The idea behind prophylactic antibiotics is that by using a small dose of medicine over a prolonged period of time, one can decrease the amount of ear infection-causing bacteria living in the nose or throat. The children on prophylactic antibiotics are still vulnerable to colds, pressure changes, and allergies that block the eustachian tube. Even if the eustachian tube is blocked, the rapid growth of bacteria necessary to produce an episode of AOM is less likely to occur.

## Which antibiotics are used?

Most of the studies showing the benefit of prophylactic antibiotics have used either amoxicillin or sulfisoxazole (Gantrisin), a sulfa drug. Trimethoprim-sulfamethoxazole (Septra, Bactrim, Sulfatrim) also is commonly used for prophylaxis, although the manufacturers recommend against this use of the drug since its safety and efficacy have not been established to Food and Drug Administration standards. (The drug has been approved for long-term prophylaxis for urinary tract infections.) The safety of repeated or prolonged use of this drug has not been established for children under the age of two for any purpose.

With the development of resistant strains of bacteria, particularly over the past two years, a wide variety of other antibiotics have been employed, although controlled studies have not yet been conducted.

Usually, prophylaxis is begun with either sulfisoxazole or amoxicillin. If these do not prove effective but prophylaxis is continued, one strategy that has met with some clinical success is to culture—by swabbing the nose and sending the specimen to a lab—to see which bacteria live in the nose and what antibiotics they are most susceptible to. Using this method, one can select a prophylactic antibiotic that is specifically geared to the most difficult to treat of the colonists of the individual child's respiratory tract. Remember: This is not treating an ear infection but trying to prevent these nasal organisms from invading the middle ear.

## What dose of an antibiotic should be given?

For prophylaxis, the appropriate dose is half the total daily dose that would be given to treat an ear infection. This is given once a day as a single dose. For prophylactic antibiotics to be successful, consistency is very important. Thus, it is a good idea to give the dose each day at bedtime since, in practice, this has been shown to promote the smallest number of missed dosages. If you do miss a night, give a dose first thing in the morning and again that evening.

## How long should prophylactic antibiotics be given?

The foundational controlled studies that demonstrated the success of prophylactic antibiotics were done using long-term daily administration. Generally, the antibiotics are continued throughout the peak AOM season—winter and early spring—for a maximum time period of about six months.

More recently, as the need to minimize antibiotic use has become increasingly clear, a number of physicians have begun using prophylactic antibiotics sporadically rather than on a continuous basis. The strategy is to give the prophylactic antibiotics daily at the first sign of an upper respiratory infection or for 72 hours before and after air travel and other high-risk exposures. This seems to work quite well. Several studies have demonstrated a decrease in the frequency of AOM by using this strategy, although the decrease is not as great as when the traditional method is used. The great advantage, though, is that by giving fewer doses of antibiotics, both the child and the community are less likely to develop severe infections with resistant bacteria.

## Do prophylactic antibiotics increase drug-resistant bacteria?

Prophylactic antibiotics have never been specifically proven to increase bacterial resistance to drugs. Margaretha Casselbrant, M.D., Ph.D., of the Otitis Media Research Center at Children's

Hospital of Pittsburgh, and colleagues (*Pediatric Infectious Disease Journal,* April 1992) performed a controlled trial in which they gave children either amoxicillin or a placebo as a prophylactic antibiotic and then checked for the presence of resistant bacteria in those children over a two-year period. In this study, there was no increase in bacterial resistance in those who received amoxicillin compared with those who received the placebo. Similar studies have not shown any increase in resistance when using sulfisoxazole as a prophylactic antibiotic.

That said, whenever an antibiotic is given, it kills the bacteria that are most susceptible to it, while the ones that are not susceptible survive. These surviving bacteria are, by definition, resistant to that antibiotic. Certainly, antibiotic use has played a role in the rapid emergence of resistant bacteria, particularly in the past two years. More recent studies have correlated the likelihood of resistant bacteria with the total amount of antibiotic a child has taken. Thus, prophylactic antibiotics should not be used indiscriminately. They should be used only for selected children with frequent ear infections—specifically, those who get quite sick with their infections, those who have speech or hearing problems, and those whose infections are so frequent that the prophylactic antibiotics might be expected to result in a smaller total dose of antibiotic over the next several months. As discussed in a previous question about frequent ear infections, this decision should be individualized and should take into account the age of the child and the time of year.

Thankfully, the vast majority of ear infections occur in the 18-month period between six months and two years of age. And only part of that time can be during the peak AOM season. Thus, the use of prophylactic antibiotics is not something that will spread out indefinitely into the future, but instead is time limited.

## What about side effects with prophylactic antibiotics?

Although side effects can occur with any antibiotic—or with any medicine, for that matter—no significant side effects occurred in any of the 15 major studies looking at either sulfisoxazole or amoxicillin as a prophylactic antibiotic (*Otitis Media in Infants and Children,* Saunders, 1995).

## How often should children on prophylactic antibiotics see their physicians?

Those children who are on prophylactic antibiotics should be examined every one to three months to assess the presence of asymptomatic OME. Management of OME is discussed below.

## What happens when my child stops taking prophylactic antibiotics?

In some studies, children who took prophylactic antibiotics experienced a honeymoon period after the antibiotics were stopped—they had fewer episodes of AOM during that period than their peers. In other studies, the rate of AOM after stopping prophylaxis returned to average for that age. There has never been a rebound effect reported, where children experience an increase in ear infections after stopping prophylactic antibiotics.

## What happens if my child gets AOM while on prophylactic antibiotics?

Prophylactic antibiotics reduce the frequency of AOM, but you should expect that ear infections will still occur, albeit less frequently. Your physician should understand that the episode of AOM that your child has is probably due to an organism that is not susceptible to the prophylactic antibiotic. Using this knowledge, an effective second-line therapy should be selected. In other words, the antibiotic choice would be the same as if the episode were a treatment failure with a first antibiotic.

Children whose track records do not adequately improve on prophylactic antibiotics should be considered as candidates for ear tubes.

## What is the correct treatment for fluid in the ear?

The second situation in which ongoing treatment decisions are necessary concerns children who have OME. Many times when a physician says that your child has an ear infection, no distinction has been made between AOM and OME. Often physicians treat all cases of otitis media the same—by prescribing antibiotics.

You will recall, however, that ear infections fall into two major categories: AOM and OME. Children with OME have fluid filling the middle ear. Children with AOM have fluid in the middle ear and signs and symptoms such as ear pain, marked redness of the eardrum, and distinct distortion of the eardrum. They often have fevers. These two different conditions call for different treatments.

Since the fluid in OME is known to contain bacteria, it came to be common practice for well-meaning physicians to prescribe antibiotics. But then in the September 15, 1993, *Journal of the American Medical Association,* an analysis of the 27 major studies looking at the treatment of OME was published. By pooling the data from all of these studies (a meta-analysis), two important conclusions were reached. First, antibiotics improve the short-term resolution of OME. Second, there is no long-term advantage to antibiotic use for OME.

In July 1994, the U.S. Department of Health and Human Services and the American Academy of Pediatrics, in concert with the American Academy of Family Physicians and the American Academy of Otolaryngology–Head and Neck Surgery, published new guidelines for managing OME in children. (Copies may be obtained by calling 800-358-9295.) These guidelines were prepared by an interdisciplinary panel of health professionals and a consumer representative.

In otherwise healthy children between the ages of one and three who have OME, the guidelines recommend environmental measures (breast-feeding, avoiding cigarette smoke, and reconsidering group day care) and either observation or antibiotics as the first-line treatment.

If the fluid is still present six weeks later, the guidelines again recommend either observation or antibiotics, with the option of a hearing evaluation.

If the child still has fluid after a total of 12 weeks, her hearing should be tested. If hearing loss is either insignificant or only in one ear, the guidelines again recommend either observation or antibiotics. (We'll discuss hearing loss in chapter 10.)

The guidelines recommend definitely treating with either antibiotics or surgical tube placement only if OME is still present after 12 weeks *and* there is hearing loss greater than 20 decibels in both ears.

If the fluid and hearing loss are still present four to six months after the initial diagnosis, the guidelines recommend tube placement. Nowhere in the guidelines are antibiotics necessarily recommended in the treatment of OME—although I would certainly try them prior to placing tubes. I would also be apt to initiate antibiotics and tubes for children with prolonged hearing loss in only one ear (see chapter 10 for the reasons why). Repeated rounds of antibiotics are difficult to justify since there is no evidence that this speeds the resolution of OME or prevents complications. Millions of cases of OME are needlessly treated with too many rounds of antibiotics.

## Are there any other ongoing treatments for OME?

A great many other ongoing treatments have been suggested for OME. The interdisciplinary team mentioned above carefully reviewed the available scientific evidence for many treatment options.

Oral steroid medications have received a lot of attention in the past few years. There is limited evidence that they do speed the resolution of OME. But as the clinical practice guidelines conclude, "The possible adverse effects (agitation, behavior change, and more serious problems such as disseminated varicella [chickenpox] in children exposed to the virus within the month before therapy) outweighed possible benefits." Steroid medications are currently not recommended for the treatment of OME in a child of any age.

Antihistamines and decongestants have been carefully studied. These medicines are not effective either separately or together for the treatment of OME. They are not recommended for this purpose in children of any age.

No recommendations were made either for or against other, more effective allergy-control measures. But it stands to reason that the child with allergies to either airborne particles or foods will benefit if these allergies are safely controlled. Reducing swelling and inflammation should give a child the optimum chance for the ear fluid to drain.

Adenoidectomy will be discussed in chapter 9. It is not recommended for isolated, uncomplicated OME in children younger than four years of age.

Tonsillectomy has been shown to be ineffective, either alone or with adenoidectomy, for the treatment of OME.

No controlled studies were found regarding chiropractic, holistic, naturopathic, traditional, indigenous, homeopathic, and other treatments. Many individuals do report cures. The same is true, however, of antihistamines, decongestants, and tonsillectomy—all of which have proven to be of no real benefit.

### ➤ *How do you treat children who have OME and AOM?*

The third situation where ongoing therapy is warranted concerns those children who have repeated acute ear infections superimposed upon chronic fluid in the ear. These children should follow the above outline for treatment of OME and should also receive antibiotics for each episode of AOM. These are the children who would likely benefit from tubes at the earlier end of the treatment spectrum.

# 9

# Surgical Therapies

## When should my child see an ear, nose, and throat (ENT) surgeon?

You should consult an ENT if your child has fluid in the middle ear for more than 12 weeks, has a hearing loss of more than 25 decibels, has recurrent episodes of acute otitis media (AOM) while on maintenance antibiotics, has a speech and language delay (in an otitis-prone child), or has one of the many possible complications of ear infections (discussed in chapter 10). Not all children who see an ENT should have surgery.

## What are ear tubes?

Called **tympanostomy tubes** or **tympanotomy tubes** because they go through the tympanic membrane (the eardrum) or PE tubes for pressure equalization, ear tubes provide a temporary, extra eustachian tube to allow bacteria and fluid to drain from the middle ear. The surgical procedure for placing tubes in the ears has become one of the most commonly performed operations of

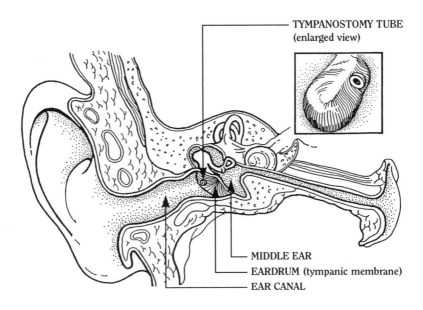

TYMPANOSTOMY TUBE
(enlarged view)

MIDDLE EAR
EARDRUM (tympanic membrane)
EAR CANAL

any kind and the most common surgery in children. The procedure is a simple one: A tiny tube with a collar on both ends (it
looks like this: ] [ and is called a **grommet** in England) is slipped
through a tiny incision in the eardrum.

In the first half of the twentieth century, it was noticed that
spontaneous holes in the eardrum often cured ear infections.
These spontaneous holes, however, appeared and closed unpre-
dictably. Several innovators tried various ways of keeping the
holes open, including inserting fish bones, lead wires, and gold
rings. Since 1954, the practice of intentionally making a small
hole in the eardrum and inserting a small tube to keep the hole
open has become very common. Today, more than 2 million ear
tubes are implanted every year in the United States (*Pediatric
Clinics of North America,* December 1996).

Ear tubes are made from a variety of materials, including
ceramic, gold, plastic, Silastic, stainless steel, Teflon, and tita-
nium. There is no proven advantage of one material over another.

## ◝ *How do tubes work?*

A tube in the eardrum improves drainage of the middle ear space. Years ago, when a can of soda was opened with a can opener, a hole was made on both sides of the lid. While fluid poured out one hole, air was able to enter the can through the other, thus improving outflow. Ear tubes function in much the same way. When the middle ear space is closed, a suction effect prevents easy clearance of the contents down the eustachian tube. A blocked eustachian tube makes this even more difficult. When a tiny hole is made in the eardrum, the contents of the middle ear space flow far more easily either down the eustachian tube or out the inserted ear tube.

Unfortunately, this can also make it easier for bacteria to enter the middle ear space. It is easier for the contents of the nose and throat to travel up the eustachian tube if there is an opening at the other end. Also, bacteria can enter through the outer ear. Studies have shown, however, that for most children, improved drainage far outweighs the increased vulnerability.

## ◝ *When are ear tubes recommended?*

In the March-April 1994 issue of the *American Journal of Otolaryngology,* respected ENT specialist Steven Handler, M.D., of Children's Hospital of Philadelphia, discussed the four generally agreed-upon indications for ear tube placement:

• First, children with prolonged otitis media with effusion (OME, or fluid in the ear) benefit from tube placement. This is the most common reason children get tubes. Tubes are often recommended after 12 weeks of OME but are occasionally recommended as early as six weeks. In some situations, which I will discuss below, waiting four to six months is appropriate.

• Second, children with recurrent AOM are candidates for tube surgery. These are children who experience at least three episodes in six months and who continue to have frequent AOM despite being placed on prophylactic antibiotics. This is the second most common reason that tubes are placed. If this recurrent AOM is mild and responds well to antibiotics, tubes are probably not necessary. On the other hand, if the child is allergic to many antibiotics, if he has severe episodes of recurrent AOM, or if the repeated bouts of AOM are having a big impact on the child or his family, the benefits of tubes outweigh the risks.

• Third, children with complicated AOM are candidates for tubes. These complications will be discussed in chapter 10. They are not common but include **abscesses**, meningitis, and facial nerve problems. An eardrum that remains hot, red, painful, and bulging despite antibiotic therapy can also be cured by tube surgery. This should not be confused with the common situation in which the child still has fluid in the ear (OME) after treatment for AOM.

• Fourth, children with complicated OME are candidates for tubes. These complications generally relate to prolonged retraction of the eardrum and its impact on the little bones of the middle ear. This is a very uncommon reason for tube placement and will be further discussed in chapter 10.

## When should early tube placement be considered?

Early tube placement should be considered for children who have any type of preexisting hearing loss or balance disorder. Children who have any other communication or sensory difficulty (visual problems, developmental delay, and so on) are also candidates for early tubes. There is no reason to delay tubes for children with known craniofacial structural problems that predispose them to recurrent infections, such as cleft palate and Down syndrome. Ongoing pain also calls for tubes at the earlier end of the spectrum. Finally, seasonal timing affects the advisability of tubes. In the fall or early winter, the child's ears are likely to get worse rather than better in the ensuing months, and early tube insertion may be warranted.

## When should tube surgery be delayed?

Some situations warrant further observation rather than a rush to tubes. Children who have OME in only one ear at a time (and who have normal language development and balance for their age) should be followed for the longer end of the spectrum. The same is true for children with bilateral OME (OME in both ears) and only mild hearing loss (less than 20 decibels). Children for whom prophylactic antibiotics result in a reduction in the frequency and/or severity of bouts of AOM also warrant further observation before ear tube placement. Tubes should be delayed for children who are less than one year old if other considerations permit. Many children experience decreases in the frequency and severity of ear infections in their second year. Finally, ear infections clear more easily and recur less readily in the spring and summer, suggesting a delay, if possible.

## Is tube surgery performed too often?

There are approximately 670,000 surgeries to insert ear tubes performed each year in the United States alone. The April 27, 1994, issue of the *Journal of the American Medical Association* contained a study of 6,429 cases of ear tube surgery. The authors' conclusion that the tubes were appropriate in only 42 percent of the cases alarmed many families who heard about the study on the news. The authors also felt that an additional 35 percent of the cases had equivocal indications (perhaps appropriate and perhaps not) and that 23 percent were inappropriate and unnecessary. This would suggest that there were more than 150,000 unnecessary tube surgeries that year, at a cost of hundreds of millions of dollars—not to mention the direct personal cost to the children and their families.

The inappropriate surgeries fell into four groups:

• Twelve percent of all tube surgeries were performed on children with frequent, recurrent AOM who had no further episodes while on prophylactic antibiotics and who had OME for less than 30 days.

• Seven percent were performed on children with recurrent (not frequent) AOM who had no episodes while on prophylactic antibiotics and who had OME for less than 30 days.

• Six percent were performed on children who had OME for less than 30 days, who were not treated with antibiotics, who had hearing loss greater than 20 decibels, and who had no recurrent AOM.

• Five percent were performed on children who had OME for less than 30 days, who were treated with antibiotics, and who had no hearing loss or recurrent AOM.

Although the paper came from the Department of Pediatrics at Harvard Medical School, the data analyzed in the paper came from Value Health Sciences, a utilization review company used by major insurance companies to cut costs and to enable them to deny certain services, including ear tube surgery. All of the authors of the paper had financial ties to Value Health Sciences as stockholders, employees, or both.

Since personal interest may subconsciously influence both sides of this issue, we must interpret the data cautiously. The "appropriate" surgeries cited in this study were certainly appropriate. The "inappropriate" surgeries may or may not have been appropriate, but further evaluation or treatment was indicated first. This may have led to resolution without surgery for many of these children.

The cases that the authors called equivocal—primarily children with frequent, recurrent AOM who continued to have infections while on prophylactic antibiotics—do have a proper surgical indication recognized by most experts in the field. I would guess that many, if not most, of the equivocal cases were actually appropriate.

Still, even if we count all of the equivocal cases as appropriate, we are left with 23 percent of tube surgeries being performed at the wrong time or on the wrong child. This is disturbing.

## If my doctor recommends tubes for my child, should I go along with it?

When surgery is suggested for your child, your responsibility as your child's guardian is to work as a partner with your physician to make a wise decision. Find out from your physician exactly what has been going on with your child. Why are tubes being recommended? Compare the story with the indications listed for tubes on pages 133–134. Has it been three weeks of AOM with a hot, red, bulging eardrum in a clearly ill child? If so, surgery and/or an antibiotic effective against resistant bacteria might be indicated. Has it been four weeks of OME in an otherwise healthy child? If so, tube surgery is not a good idea.

Parents can have mixed feelings when a doctor suggests surgery for their child. Finally, a light appears at the end of the antibiotic tunnel. There's hope for uninterrupted sleep. But maybe you don't want your little one to have surgery. And then if the pediatrician and the surgeon disagree about what to do, the whole situation becomes very unsettling. Equipped with the information in this book, you can be not a blind follower but an informed partner in the care of your child.

## How long do tubes remain in the ears?

Most ear tubes spontaneously fall out as the eardrum grows. On average, this occurs between six and 12 months after surgery, although in many children the tubes can remain in place for years. The interval in which the tubes are in place is usually enough to carry a child through one peak season of AOM. The hope is that after this time, the child will have grown enough to make further infections less likely. There are permanent tubes that are sometimes put in children's ears. Usually, this should not be done unless the child has some permanent abnormality causing eustachian tube dysfunction (such as Down syndrome).

## When should ear tubes be removed?

For the great majority of children, the tubes should be allowed to spontaneously exit. Since tube removal is usually done under general anesthesia, it is desirable to delay the procedure until it becomes probable that the tube won't come out on its own and the child is old enough that he is very unlikely to need another set of tubes. There is no exact consensus on the timing of tube removal. Most children are very unlikely to have further ear infections once they reach age six. Therefore, tubes are generally removed when a child makes it through kindergarten without further ear infections. Removal may be done at an earlier age if the child has one tube in place and one intact eardrum, provided the intact eardrum has no evidence of infection for a one-year period. Tubes may also be removed earlier if the child is having a problem with the tubes, such as chronic **otorrhea**, or drainage from the ear.

## How much do ear tubes cost?

When my son had tubes placed in 1996, the hospital costs were as follows:

| Service Description | Quantity | Charges ($) | Total Charges ($) |
|---|---|---|---|
| Microscope use | 1 | 84.50 | 84.50 |
| Surgery gloves | 2 | 14.50 | 29.00 |
| Surgical instrument use | 1 | 81.30 | 81.30 |
| Blade (disposable) | 1 | 30.70 | 30.70 |
| Short-stay surgery— operating room time | 15 min. | 61.95/min | 929.25 |
| Ear tube | 2 | 112.25 | 224.50 |
| Suction tubing—6 feet | 1 | 4.75 | 4.75 |
| **Total Operating Room** | | | **1,384.00** |
| Recovery room time | 30 min. | 8.86/min | 265.70 |
| **Total Recovery Room** | | | **265.70** |
| Sensor pad | 1 | 87.75 | 87.75 |
| Stethoscope | 1 | 29.50 | 29.50 |
| General anesthesia | 45 min. | 10.42/min | 469.00 |
| Syringe | 1 | 4.75 | 4.75 |
| EKG monitor use | 1 | 20.05 | 20.05 |
| Blood pressure monitor use | 1 | 9.25 | 9.25 |
| Oxygen saturation monitor use | 1 | 24.80 | 24.80 |
| Anesthesia breathing tube | 1 | 17.75 | 17.75 |
| Mask—adult king-size | 1 | 17.50 | 17.50 |
| Mask—bubble gum* | 1 | 28.25 | 28.25 |
| Needle | 1 | 11.00 | 11.00 |
| **Total Anesthesia** | | | **719.60** |
| Pediatric preoperative care | 60 min. | 230.00 | 230.00 |
| Pediatric recovery care | 60 min. | 1.17/min. | 70.20 |
| **Total Pediatrics** | | | **300.20** |
| Cortisporin eardrops | 1 | 32.10 | 32.10 |
| Ibuprofen | 1 | 27.60 | 27.60 |
| **Total Pharmacy** | | | **59.70** |
| **TOTAL HOSPITAL CHARGES** | | | **2,729.20** |

*This mask, used in anesthetizing children, emits a pleasant bubble-gum scent to help children fall asleep.

These fees are for a community hospital in California and may not be the same in other areas and in other types of hospitals.

The ear, nose, and throat surgeon and the anesthesiologist bill separately from the hospital costs. In my area, a surgeon charges about $1,200 on average, and an anesthesiologist charges about $500. This brings the grand total for the 15-minute procedure to approximately $4,400.

## What are the risks of ear tube placement?

Parents' major concern about ear tube placement is the risk of general anesthesia. Ear tube surgery is very quick, lasting a total of only 10 to 15 minutes, and would be expected to have a minimal anesthesia risk. One study done by L. Markowitz-Spence, of the State University of New York, Buffalo School of Medicine, published in the July 1990 *Archives of Otolaryngology–Head and Neck Surgery,* looked at 510 children who had tubes placed and found no serious complications or deaths. This is somewhat reassuring, but the numbers are too small to uncover potential risks.

The biggest risk of such a short operation is a severe allergic reaction to the general anesthesia. Overall, this occurs in about one of every 10,000 operations. Between 0.1 percent and 5 percent of those who have these severe reactions die. (That's one death for every 200,000 to 10,000,000 operations.)

## Do tubes decrease hearing?

Although children with tubes in place usually hear normally, tube-containing eardrums are slightly less sensitive to sound than normal eardrums. The choice, though, is not between a healthy ear and one with tubes but between a chronically infected ear and one with tubes. Since tubes are usually put into fluid-filled ears, the short-term effect is to improve hearing. The goal of tube surgery, in fact, is to protect hearing—particularly during times of rapid learning.

## What is the long-term effect of tubes on hearing?

The great majority of children who have ear tubes will experience no long-term effect on their hearing. Some will have hearing loss.

Researchers at the University of Rochester Medical Center undertook a study to determine the long-term effect of tubes on hearing. They looked at 43 children (or 86 ears) who had each received at least three sets of ear tubes. They compared them with 46 children (or 92 ears) who had frequent, severe ear infections (1,334 ear infections in these 46 children). This group received antibiotics alone. Abnormal hearing was found in 9 to 18 percent of the ears that had at least three operations but only 4 to 9 percent of the ears treated without surgery. The difference between the two groups was 5 to 9 percent. Thus, repeated tube surgeries do cause hearing loss in a relatively small percentage of children (*Pediatric Infectious Disease Journal,* November 1989).

Most children with tubes have normal hearing, even if there is scarring of the eardrum (see below). The more ear infections and the more operations a child has, however, the greater the likelihood that hearing will be compromised.

## What other complications are there?

The most common complication is scarring of the eardrum (**tympanosclerosis**). This scarring can occur both from frequent or prolonged otitis media and from ear tube insertion. It turns out that the scarring is about 50 percent more common in children who have the tubes placed than in matched children who use other therapies. Thankfully, the scarring generally doesn't affect anything but appearance—and not that many people will be looking inside your child's ear.

Another problem that can occur after the tubes spontaneously leave is that a perforation, or hole, can be left in the eardrum. This occurs in about 15 percent of children, but most of the holes close on their own. Between 1 and 2 percent of children with tubes eventually need surgery to close the hole.

## What's it like to have tubes put in?

If you are considering tubes for your child, I'm sure that he has had a long and difficult battle with ear infections. Like most parents, you probably aren't eager to have your young child go through a surgical procedure. But you are faced with an ongoing battle that may include continuous antibiotic use, possible hearing loss, and lack of sleep (for the entire family). By the time most parents decide to have the procedure done, they are physically and emotionally very worn out. I know we were!

At this point, your child's primary care physician will refer your child to an ear, nose, and throat (ENT) surgeon. If you have managed care insurance, the ENT must be approved by your insurance plan. This may or may not be the doctor that you would prefer, but managed care saves money by limiting choices.

During your first visit to the ENT, she will review your child's medical history and perform a physical exam before making a recommendation. More often than not, if a child has gotten to this point, an ENT will recommend the surgery.

The surgery is then scheduled, pending insurance approval if needed. HMOs and some other types of plans require preapproval. Some traditional indemnity insurance plans do not require preapproval. The length of time until the surgery will be determined by your ENT's schedule, how booked the hospital operating room is, and how long it takes to get approval from your insurance plan. All of this generally takes a few weeks.

The ENT who will be performing surgery on your child may have privileges at one or more hospitals. If she has privileges at only one hospital, then you will be forced to have the surgery at that hospital. If she practices at more than one hospital, you may have some say in the choice of hospitals, although your insurance plan may only cover the cost of the procedure at a particular hospital. Your ENT's office should help you to sort through these details.

A few days before the surgery, you will need to register with the hospital admissions staff. This is generally done during business hours and can be done by phone at some hospitals.

The day before the surgery, you will be given a surgery time. Plan to take the entire day off work. In most hospitals, tube surgeries are done early in the day. But even if that's not the case for you, you will want to be home with your child, who is not allowed to eat or drink anything for eight hours before the surgery.

## What should I expect on the day of the surgery?

On the day of the surgery, plan to check in about two hours in advance. It is important that you arrive at the time the hospital tells you to. At some hospitals, surgeries are canceled if the patient is 15 minutes late! After you check in, a nurse will walk you through some paperwork and take your child's vital signs. You will be given a hospital gown to put on your child and shown to a space where you can wait (usually you get a room with a bed, but not always). You and your child will spend most of the next two hours waiting. Your child won't have eaten in at least eight hours and will be ready for food. He will be aware that something out of the ordinary is happening. As the time wears on, your child will probably become more anxious (and more hungry). Often the surgery is not started at the scheduled time, so you may have to wait even longer than the two interminable hours that you had already planned on waiting.

Finally, the anesthesiologist will come to talk with you. She will explain what medications your child will have during surgery. By this time, your child will probably be feeling very scared. He will sense that "something bad" is going to happen, and you might have some trouble consoling him. If your child is going through separation anxiety, he will probably be very clingy. If your child is a bit older and tends to express apprehension through acting out, he will probably be difficult to control. These behaviors are only natural. Do not be concerned about what the people around you may think. Try to comfort him in whatever way works. If your child is clingy, then by all means hold him. If your child is being physical, then engage him in a physical game. This is a very important time for your child.

After what seems like an eternity, someone will come to take you to the surgical area. You may be able to carry your child, or they may ask you to put him on a rolling bed. You should be able to accompany your child to the surgical area. When you arrive, you will be asked to stay in the waiting room. The staff will most likely be very accustomed to working with children and will treat your child with great care and tenderness. Still, your child may come unglued when he has to leave you.

It's a good thing that tube surgery is very brief.

During the next 30 to 45 minutes, you will probably come close to wearing out a spot on the carpet outside the waiting room. I know I did. As much as I know about medicine and as familiar as I am with hospitals, I still find it difficult to watch someone I love being wheeled away into surgery. I know the risks of general anesthesia are very, very small, but I still feel better when I know my loved one is safely recovering.

As soon as your child is wheeled into the operating room, he is anesthetized, usually by breathing gas through a mask. Your child will not remember anything from this point on until he is in the recovery room.

The surgical procedure is very simple. A small incision is made in the eardrum, and the tube is inserted. Any pus or fluid is drained from the middle ear at this time, and antibiotic drops are placed in the ear. The procedure itself takes only minutes. Following the surgery, the surgeon should come out to speak with you. She will tell you how the surgery went and give you instructions to follow over the next few days.

Immediately following the surgery, your child will be moved to the recovery room, where he will be observed until fully awake (your child will be somewhat groggy for another few hours). Your child will be waking up in a strange room from a very deep sleep. It is not uncommon for a child in this situation to be frightened.

When your child has recovered from the effects of the sedation, he will be taken to a hospital room, where you must stay until he recovers enough to eat. You may stay in the hospital room for as long as two hours before you are released to go home. During this time, your child may be afraid of what is going to happen next. He will undoubtedly want to be held and reassured.

Your child may not be his normal self for the rest of the day. But as soon as the anesthesia fully wears off and he eats something, he will begin to feel much better.

When most parents look back at the whole experience a few weeks afterward, the event seems much smaller and less traumatic than they had anticipated.

## Can parents join their children in the recovery room?

When my son had ear tubes placed, I was not allowed to be with him in the recovery room as he woke up—restrained, in a strange place, surrounded by strangers who needed to examine him. He was 10 months old, at the peak of separation anxiety and stranger anxiety. I was stunned that this could happen. I was trained in a children's hospital where this would never have happened.

Whether you are allowed in the recovery room depends on the hospital. Many hospitals, especially children's hospitals, encourage parents to be present when their child wakes up from general anesthesia. However, many hospitals still cling to the tradition of refusing to admit parents into the recovery room. They cite issues of privacy for other recovering patients and interruptions of recovery room procedures. I think this antiquated, authoritarian practice should be stopped.

Not many decades ago, parents were told not to even visit their children if they were admitted to the hospital. Thankfully, we have realized that this policy is a terrible mistake. Today, having a parent room-in with a child is the norm in most hospitals. Not surprisingly, studies have shown that this practice benefits everybody.

Whenever studies have focused on the presence of parents in the recovery room, they have likewise shown that this significantly benefited both the children and the parents (*Pediatric Alert,* February 1996). Each year, evidence continues to mount that in most situations both children and parents do better if the parents are present and involved with their children's care.

If one of my children needs surgery again, I plan to inquire about each hospital's policy in this regard prior to deciding which hospital to use. I hope that the hospital administration would rather bend its outdated policy than lose the business. If not, then perhaps if enough parents do the same, hospitals will decide to abandon this archaic practice altogether.

### How do I prepare my child for surgery?

The answer to this depends on both the age of your child and your child's personality. Fears about what might happen next usually are far worse than the actual event. This can be helped by letting your child know what to expect. This might include verbally telling the child the step-by-step itinerary. It might include watching a video provided by your hospital. You might make up an ear tube game to play with your child, pretending to put an ear tube in a favorite stuffed animal to make its ear stop hurting. You might want to plan a visit to the hospital (especially the cafeteria), so you can have fun there together beforehand.

Whatever your child's age and personality, it is valuable for you to take a few minutes beforehand to try to put yourself in your child's shoes. Walk through each step of the journey ahead. Your empathy will make a big difference.

### Will my child's ear be better immediately afterward?

Hopefully. Somewhere between 12 and 15 percent of children have drainage out of the ear tubes in the days immediately following the ear surgery. For the past several years, antibiotic eardrops have been used for several days after surgery. This has been effective in somewhat decreasing the rate of ear drainage.

### Are antibiotic eardrops safe?

The antibiotics contained in eardrops are drugs known to cause ear damage in some children when taken intravenously. Do they cause damage when applied directly to the ear? A prospective, randomized study of the safety of topical eardrops was published in the May 1995 issue of *Laryngoscope*. Fifty children with bilateral tubes had antibiotic drops placed in one ear. One child had mild hearing loss, but it was the same in the treated and the untreated ears. No other untoward effect was found.

In a larger study from University Hospital in Zurich, Switzerland (*American Journal of Otology,* September 1995), the authors reviewed all of the patient charts from 1953 to the present, looking for ear damage possibly related to topical eardrops. They found two patients who had profound hearing loss, and both had been taking prolonged, excessive antibiotic drops.

Intermittent, short courses of these drops appear to be quite safe, but they should not be used indiscriminately. Parents often wind up with a supply at home and then use them without the doctor knowing the usage pattern. Be very clear on how and when your doctor wants you to use them. If your child seems to be in pain when they are administered, be sure to report this to your doctor before any further use.

## Are there any recent innovations in ear tubes?

Recently, some surgeons have been using ear tubes impregnated with silver oxide in an effort to decrease the number of infected or draining ears after tube insertion. Silver oxide is an active compound made from silver and oxygen. It can oxidize, or give oxygen to, other materials that it touches. It is commonly used in watch batteries. Silver oxide is known to inhibit the growth of bacteria. In a multicenter, double-blind, randomized clinical trial, published in the May 1995 *Archives of Otolaryngology–Head and Neck Surgery,* the use of the new silver oxide tubes cut the overall incidence of draining or infected ears by almost half during the year following surgery (from 9.78 percent with the traditional tubes to 5.08 percent with the new tubes). There were no increased side effects with the silver oxide tubes.

## How do you treat AOM with ear tubes in place?

One of the advantages of the ear tubes is that when AOM is present, you will know by a purulent drainage coming from the ear. Another advantage is that the infection is usually easier to clear. The infection can be treated with oral and/or topical antibiotics.

If the infection does not easily clear, the fluid draining from the ear can be sent to a lab for analysis to indicate the ideal antibiotic for the infection.

### ➤ What do you do for frequently recurrent AOM in a child with tubes?

When you proceed all the way to ear tubes, it is very disappointing to still have frequently recurrent ear infections. Before you treat the infection, it is important to find out why it's occurring. It is not unusual to have an occasional ear infection with ear tubes; about half of children have at least one episode in the three years following tube placement. But frequently recurrent episodes are very uncommon. The most likely cause is a blocked ear tube. The tiny tube opening can be obstructed by a drop of blood, mucus, or another secretion. Your doctor should get a good view of the tube to see if it is blocked or falling out.

### ➤ What do you do if the ear tube gets blocked?

In the March 1995 issue of the *International Journal of Pediatric Otorhinolaryngology,* physicians at the Royal Ear Hospital in London reported their experience with two different types of eardrops for clearing blocked ear tubes. They compared sodium bicarbonate eardrops with hydrogen peroxide eardrops in a randomized, controlled trial. The drops were equally effective, and both were more effective than any period of observation alone. If the ear tubes do not open with two weeks of treatment, surgical replacement should be considered.

### ➤ How do you treat frequently recurrent AOM in a child with open, functioning ear tubes?

This uncommon and discouraging situation should be treated the same way as frequently recurrent AOM in a child without tubes.

## Are most parents glad that their children have had tube surgery?

Most parents of children who have had ear tubes placed are happy with the results. They report fewer ear infections, easier clearance when infections do occur, and less worrying about whether their children have ear infections. Most children are happier, and they're sick less often. A study published in the October 1996 *Laryngoscope* reported that 93 percent of parents were satisfied overall with the results of the operation and that 87 percent of parents would want the surgery again if another of their children were to develop similar problems.

Another recent study showed that ear tubes improve not only children's ear infections and hearing but also their behavior and overall quality of life. Melissa Wake, M.D., of the Royal Children's Hospital in Melbourne, Australia, reported the results of her well-designed, controlled study at the 1996 annual meeting of the Pediatric Academic Societies. She found some surprising and dramatic benefits for those children who had tubes. Their parents noticed that the children became healthier in general than those in the study who did not receive tubes. The parents also noticed that the children who received tubes developed longer attention spans, were happier with themselves, spoke more quietly, were better behaved, no longer had bad breath, and had less nasal stuffiness and discharge. Thus, the surgery benefited not only the children's physical health but also their relationships with others.

For many parents, the most vexing issue is the need for water precautions. Neither making their children wear earplugs nor limiting water exposure is very fun.

## Should a child swim with ear tubes?

Here is a sample of the many questions I get on this subject:

Dr. Greene,

My four-year-old son recently had ear tubes placed. My doctor said that it is okay for him to go swimming (I think). My friends look at me horrified. They say he needs to wear custom earplugs. Their doctors told them that their children with ear tubes shouldn't let their ears get wet. My son loves the water. What should I do?

*Scottsdale, Arizona*

For years, ear, nose, and throat specialists cautioned against allowing water in an ear that has an open tube in the eardrum. Recently, some have begun to suggest that swimming precautions are unnecessary—that water does not get through the tiny tube into the middle ear. Over the past few years, there has been a flurry of articles arguing both points of view. This controversy has led to a good deal of confusion among parents.

Thankfully, it's okay for most children with ear tubes to swim without earplugs. An excellent study was published in the March 1996 *Archives of Otolaryngology–Head and Neck Surgery* that may finally end this controversy. The investigators followed 399 children with ear tubes. The children were divided into four groups at the beginning of the study. Children in the first group were encouraged to swim without precautions. Those in the second group received antibiotic eardrops each night after they had been in the water. Those in the third group wore molded earplugs whenever they were in the water. Children in all three of these groups were instructed against diving and swimming more than six feet beneath the surface (since water under pressure presumably enters the middle ear through the tiny tubes more readily). The fourth group consisted of confirmed nonswimmers. All parents were warned not to allow soapy water to enter the ears during bathing since the lower surface tension of soapy water could allow it to penetrate the tubes more easily. Also, soapy water could be more irritating to the middle ear if it gains entrance.

Children in the three groups of swimmers showed no inter-group difference in the incidence of ear infections or draining ears, regardless of plugs or eardrops. There was also no difference between the swimmers and nonswimmers. This study, however, looked only at swimming in swimming pools. Lake, pond, and river water as well as bathwater may all contain more bacteria than pool water. Thus, for the time being, caution is wise in the nonpool venues.

The conclusion: Let your child enjoy swimming in the pool. Forget earplugs. If your child turns out to be one of the unfortunate few who gets frequent ear infections in the summer months even after tubes, you might want to try water precautions on the chance that he is particularly sensitive to water exposure.

Perhaps sometime soon, someone will do a study of whether diving, underwater swimming, pond water, and soapy bathwater precautions are all really necessary. In the meantime, better safe than sorry.

## Is adenoidectomy ever done for ear infections?

Adenoidectomy, or removal of the adenoid glands, is a common major surgical procedure that is used to prevent recurrent ear infections. Adenoidectomy with or without tonsillectomy is the most common major operation performed in the United States, accounting for about half of all major operations performed on children.

## When should adenoidectomy be considered?

Adenoidectomy is a particularly useful option for children three years of age and older. These children are more likely to benefit from adenoid surgery, while children younger than three are more likely to have complications from this surgery. When surgery is considered for the prevention of otitis media, I usually recommend ear tube insertion alone, unless there is a compelling reason to also perform an adenoidectomy, such as significant obstruction at the back of the nose by the adenoid glands. There is an increased likelihood that the adenoids are obstructing the opening of the eustachian tube if your child snores, mouth-breathes and snores, has chronic nasal congestion and snores, or is more than three or four years old with continued ear infections.

When a child has a resurgence of ear infections after the initial tubes have exited, then I usually recommend adenoidectomy at the same time as other tubes are inserted.

There have been a great many studies looking at the benefits and risks of adenoidectomies, and they have had conflicting results. A very well designed study by J.L. Paradise, M.D., of the University of Pittsburgh School of Medicine, and colleagues, published in the April 1990 *Journal of the American Medical Association,* did show a clear but modest benefit from this procedure in children who had previously had ear tubes placed and who continued to have infections after the tubes had fallen out.

## ➤ *When should tonsillectomy be considered?*

On November 26, 1983, the *British Medical Journal* reported a large study by A. Richard Maw, M.D., consulting ear, nose, and throat specialist of the British Royal Infirmary, in which he analyzed the benefits of adenoidectomy with or without tonsillectomy. There was no difference in the progress of middle ear disease between children who did or did not have their tonsils removed. At present, there is no evidence that tonsillectomy is of any benefit in the treatment or prevention of otitis media. I would recommend tonsillectomy only for a child who has frequent ear infections—and only if he has some other concurrent condition that makes tonsillectomy otherwise compelling, such as obstruction of the airway or sleep apnea.

# 10

# Complications

## ⌒ *Does antibiotic use affect complications?*

Before antibiotics were in common use for the treatment of otitis media, serious complications were relatively common. Today, serious complications are relatively uncommon. In fact, the rate of serious complications is more than 200 times lower when antibiotics are commonly used. In some places where antibiotic use for otitis media was discouraged (such as Germany), the complication rate has increased again (*Pediatrics,* October 1995). Thus, although about two-thirds of children would get better without any antibiotics whatsoever, it is important either to treat children who have otitis media with antibiotics or to follow them very closely to prevent the serious complications that will be discussed in this chapter.

## ⌒ *Do all ear infections cause hearing loss?*

Both acute otitis media (AOM) and otitis media with effusion (OME) are accompanied by fluid in the middle ear. Whenever fluid is present in the middle ear space, hearing is impaired. Hearing loss is the most prevalent complication of OME. Children with recurrent episodes of otitis media or with persistent middle ear fluid perform more poorly on tests of speech and language than other children of the same age who have clear ears. The fluid in the ear causes a **conductive hearing loss**, meaning that sound is poorly conducted across the middle ear space. This results in a muffling of about 15 to 40 decibels. These children can still hear, but some of the softer speech sounds may be missed entirely. To give you an idea of what this means, absolute silence is 0 decibels; an empty recording studio has a background sound of 20 decibels; a quiet room in a home has a background sound of 40 decibels; and a normal conversation is 60 decibels. A 15-decibel hearing loss would make a conversation sound as if it were being overheard from another table in a busy restaurant— many details would be missed.

## Does the type of fluid influence the degree of hearing loss?

People are often told that short-term fluid in the ear is thin and produces a mild hearing loss, whereas fluid that remains for a long time becomes thick and produces a greater hearing loss. This is not the case.

Thin, straw-colored, watery fluid and thick, viscous, gluelike fluid cause essentially identical hearing loss. Any fluid behind the eardrum has a density so much greater than air that sound waves are reflected off of the eardrum rather than proceeding through the middle ear.

## What does determine the amount of hearing loss?

The most important determinant of hearing loss is the volume of fluid present in the middle ear. The more space that is taken up by fluid, the less mobility the eardrum has, and the poorer a child's hearing will be. Conversely, the more air that remains, the better hearing will be.

## How can I know how much hearing loss is present?

The degree of hearing loss can be measured with an audiometer. This should be done in children with prolonged fluid in the ears and in children who have any speech delay, as discussed in chapter 5.

Some clues to the degree of hearing loss are also available on physical examination. Since ears that are only partially filled with fluid conduct sound better than ears that are completely filled, one can look for evidence of remaining air. When bubbles or an air-fluid level is visible beyond the eardrum, there is still some air in the middle ear space. Clearly, the presence of fluid in both ears is much more damaging than when the fluid is present in only one ear. Generally, hearing is restored when the fluid disappears.

## Is permanent hearing loss a problem with otitis media?

Most of the hearing loss associated with otitis media is a conductive hearing loss that resolves when the fluid disappears. Occasionally, however, conductive hearing loss can become permanent when the fluid damages the middle ear space or the tiny bones of the middle ear. In addition, otitis media can cause **sensorineural hearing loss**—hearing loss associated with damage to the cochlea. Reversible sensory hearing loss occurs from pressure on the round window of the cochlea. This resolves when the fluid in the middle ear disappears. On occasion, bacteria, viruses, enzymes, neurotoxins, and other chemicals can cross the round window and invade the inner ear. This results in permanent hearing loss.

## When should children be referred for a hearing test?

If you think you notice that your child has hearing loss, an audiologic evaluation is indicated. Parents are often the first to suspect such a problem. A hearing test is also important if your child has any speech or language delay. Even if your child has no signs or symptoms of hearing loss, her hearing should be tested if fluid is present for 12 weeks.

## What is speech or language delay?

On average, a child begins cooing by about two months of age and making single vowel sounds by three months of age. Laughing out loud begins at about four months; babbling, at six months. Repetitive consonant sounds (*mamama, dadada*) emerge at about 10 months. The first word (the same sound used for the same person or object) is usually spoken at about 12 months.

An average 15-month old uses four to six words plus a great deal of jargon. The ability to follow simple requests is expected at this age.

A typical 18-month old has about 10 words and can identify one or more parts of the body. By 19 months, she is putting two words together in a phrase ("Mommy drink").

By age two, an average child puts three words together (subject-verb-object) and has a vocabulary of 50 to 100 words or more. Two-step requests can be understood and followed.

The greatest development of vocabulary occurs between ages two and five. A child goes from 50 to 100 words to more than 2,000. Speech should be clearly understandable by age three.

There is a wide normal variation in language development. Still, any child who meets one of the following criteria, adapted from the *Nelson Textbook of Pediatrics* (Saunders, 1996), should be referred for audiologic testing:

- *12 months:* no babbling or vocal imitation
- *18 months:* no use of single words
- *24 months:* vocabulary of 10 words or less
- *30 months:* vocabulary of less than 100 words, no two-word phrases
- *36 months:* vocabulary of less than 200 words, no sentences, clarity of less than 50 percent
- *48 months:* vocabulary of less than 600 words, no complete sentences, clarity of less than 80 percent

## Do frequent ear infections affect normal childhood development?

Language development during the first few years of life is nothing short of amazing. A child is born unable to understand any words yet is speaking in complete sentences within a few years. During this flowering of development, there are certain critical windows when different sounds are learned. It has been established that children who grow up not hearing particular sounds may not be able to distinguish them later. Thus, someone who reaches eight to 10 months of age without hearing Chinese will lose the ability to distinguish between some of the vocal sounds of that language.

What a tragedy if the language you miss out on hearing is your own! The time when the miracle of language development is unfolding is the same time when children most frequently get ear infections. Chronic ear infections do result in measurable language delays. It stands to reason that hearing loss could disrupt or delay language development, which could in turn lead to poor speech, which could decrease communication and slow the child in every area of intellectual and social development. But this line of reasoning contains many suppositions.

A great many studies have been undertaken to try to estimate the magnitude of the effect, if any, of ear infections on childhood development. Unfortunately, these studies are very hard to control scientifically since the critical window for learning a particular sound may come at different ages from one child to the next. Also, other variables such as the presence of day care, the way the family interacts with the child, and the time in which one (or two) ears are involved in ear infections all tend to confound the results. In a conversation I had with Robert Ruben, M.D., of Albert Einstein College of Medicine, he spoke with great passion as he described a group of children he has followed for the past nine years. They all had fluid in the ears for at least 30 percent of the time between six and 12 months of age. They still have measurable language delays nine years later! Ruben says he couldn't perform this test again since it would be immoral to let children continue this long with fluid in their ears now that we know the long-term consequences.

A large independent study from Finland found that children who had more than four episodes of AOM before their third birthdays were measurably poorer readers at nine years of age than their counterparts (*Pediatric Infectious Disease Journal,* October 1996).

Evidence is mounting that chronic and recurrent ear infections do indeed have an impact on language development and on development in general. The American Academy of Pediatrics has issued a policy statement saying that "there is growing evidence demonstrating a correlation between middle ear disease, hearing impairment, and the delays in development of speech, language, and cognitive skills." This possibility underscores the need to treat each individual child optimally. Fluid in the ear should be followed closely until it resolves. Children with prolonged fluid in the ear should have their hearing tested, and their development should be followed particularly closely. Don't let your child fall through the cracks of the medical system.

## Do children with hearing loss in only one ear have developmental consequences?

While most people think that hearing well in one ear permits normal development, research conducted at the Bill Wilkerson Hearing and Speech Center in Tennessee has shown that this is not true. Fred Bess, Ph.D., and colleagues published a series of papers in issues of *Pediatrics* and *Ear and Hearing* from 1986 to 1995 that demonstrate measurable developmental consequences, including an increased rate of school failure among children with unilateral hearing loss (in one ear only) compared with children with normal hearing. This difference is greater for boys than for girls and for hearing loss in the right ear than for hearing loss in the left ear. Sounds reaching the right ear should be processed by the left brain, where the primary speech center is located. Girls tend to have more connections between the two sides of the brain than boys, thus protecting them from the worst consequences of unilateral hearing loss. These findings make me more likely to recommend ear tubes for a child with prolonged fluid in the ear, even if the hearing loss is unilateral.

## Could you tell me about perforation of the eardrum?

In some children, the pressure inside the middle ear space is so great that the eardrum spontaneously ruptures and a small, or even large, hole in the eardrum opens. In some groups of children (Eskimos and some Native American tribes), the eardrum is perforated with almost every episode of AOM. Some children not in these high-risk groups have similar patterns. Most cases of perforation occur sporadically, due to rapidly multiplying bacteria in a completely sealed cavity.

## ➤ Does the perforation make the infection worse?

The perforation allows the infected fluid to drain out of the ear. The discharge is visible, dripping out of the ear canal. The opening also allows the infected fluid in the ear to leave more easily via the eustachian tube, in the same way that the soda can once needed two openings (one to allow soda to get out and the other to allow air to get in).

Children with perforated eardrums should be placed on an oral antibiotic just like children with AOM. Some physicians also advocate putting antibiotic drops directly into the ear. This usually speeds resolution of the infection, but it is often not necessary since the infection itself is often easier to clear once a perforation has occurred.

Since the eardrum is perforated and the infected contents are present in the external ear canal, a physician can obtain a small amount of the fluid and send it to a laboratory for culture. This makes it possible to determine exactly which bacteria are causing the particular infection and to be certain that the actual bacteria in the ear are susceptible to the chosen antibiotic. Culturing the ear and using topical antibiotic drops are particularly important if the ear infection does not quickly clear after perforation.

## ➤ Does a perforation hurt?

Children typically experience intense ear pain before the eardrum ruptures. This ear pain comes from the stretching of the eardrum. Once the rupture occurs, the child may no longer complain of pain at all.

If the child has persistent pain following a perforation, one should suspect another complication, such as mastoiditis (see page 167). This is particularly true if the ear or the area immediately behind it is swollen or red or feels tender to the touch.

A CAT scan (computer-enhanced cross-sectional x-ray image) of the head may help to pinpoint the location of this infection.

If a discharge of pus continues for two to three weeks without responding to treatment, the child should be hospitalized for intensive evaluation and treatment—even if she has no other symptoms.

In most cases of perforation of the eardrum, however, the ear infection clears relatively quickly, and the perforation closes within a week after the infection is gone.

## ➤ *What if the perforation doesn't close?*

In some children, a hole in the eardrum may persist. If the hole is there longer than two months without signs of infection, this is called a chronic perforation.

There are advantages and disadvantages to a chronic perforation. The chronic perforation can in many ways act like ear tubes that have been surgically installed. The perforation can actually prevent infections and can make infections, when they do occur, far easier to treat. Thus, treatment of a small, uncomplicated chronic hole in the eardrum is often delayed until the child is beyond the age of frequent ear infections. Generally, this surgery is delayed until at least age six or seven.

There are also problems associated with a chronic perforation, however. By itself, a perforation of the eardrum does result in some hearing loss. A small perforation (like ear tubes) generally results in insignificant hearing loss. The hearing is, in fact, often improved if the child previously had fluid in the ear. However, a moderate to large perforation can result in a significant hearing loss in the 20- to 40-decibel range—enough to affect hearing and development.

Also, in the same way that a hole in the eardrum can make it easier for fluid in the eardrum to drain, a hole in the eardrum makes it easier for bacteria and other fluid to enter the eardrum.

When the eardrum is intact and the middle ear space is a closed cavity, it is difficult for the contents of the nose and throat to make their way through the eustachian tube and up into the middle ear space. When a hole is present in the eardrum (either a perforation or a tube), the contents of the nose and throat are not as effectively blocked. Thus, some children with perforation have an increased number of episodes of recurrent AOM.

As if this weren't enough, if the hole in the eardrum is large enough, it may allow contaminated water to enter the middle ear from the outside, particularly during bathing and swimming.

The overall effect of the perforation depends on the size and location of the hole, as well as the anatomy and immune status of the child. Thus, the decision of when to close a chronic perforation needs to be made based on the situation of each individual child.

When possible, the procedure should be delayed until after age seven to maximize the safety and efficacy of the surgery. In some children, hearing loss or stubborn ear infections may make early closure a better option.

Eardrum repair (or tympanoplasty) is a common surgery in children.

### What is chronic purulent otitis media?

Some children have ear infections that result in a perforation of the eardrum that continues to drain pus over a long period of time. This condition, called **chronic purulent otitis media**, is much more difficult to treat than either AOM or OME. It is often associated with other complications, such as mastoiditis and cholesteatoma (see page 165). Chronic purulent otitis media occurs when bacteria that normally live in the external ear canal travel through a perforated eardrum and set up residence in the middle ear space. These bacteria are quite different from the ones generally found in other types of ear infections. The most common species of bacteria is called *Pseudomonas aeruginosa*. This is followed by *Staphylococcus aureus* and diphtheroids. Together, these account for more than half of the cases of chronic purulent otitis media. There are at least 20 different species of bacteria that account for the other half of cases.

### ➤ How is chronic purulent otitis media treated?

The bacteria that cause chronic purulent otitis media do not respond well to the oral antibiotics used for the treatment of AOM. Some respond to topical antibiotic drops such as Cortisporin and gentamycin. Some, however, require therapy with one or more intravenous antibiotics. Children with chronic purulent otitis media are at the highest risk for developing further complications and may require immediate surgery.

### ➤ What is a cholesteatoma?

Cholesteatomas are nothing more than accumulations of old skin cells. Nevertheless, they are among the most dreaded complications of ear infections.

A cholesteatoma begins when a small portion of the eardrum is pulled in to form a retraction pocket or pouch. This may look like a perforation. The small sack of eardrum begins to accumulate dead skin cells. The sack enlarges and begins to erode the tiny bones of the middle ear. The cholesteatoma behaves like a tumor, eroding the bones of the skull and destroying tissue as it grows. It can cause facial paralysis by destroying the facial nerve. The growing mass of dead skin cells can cause meningitis and infections of the brain. These severe infections and the direct brain damage can cause death in children.

Before antibiotics were used to treat ear infections, cholesteatomas were common. The complications of cholesteatomas were also common. A great many children died from cholesteatomas following ear infections. Today, cholesteatomas are far less common, occurring in somewhere around six of every 100,000 children.

## ➤ How is a cholesteatoma diagnosed?

Unfortunately, a cholesteatoma is a silent complication. The child frequently has no complaint. Adults with cholesteatomas usually describe fullness in the ear, ringing in the ear, or **vertigo** (dizziness). Children typically do not describe these symptoms, either because they are not aware of them or because they are too young to describe them. By the time symptoms such as facial paralysis, severe headache, vomiting, and severe vertigo occur, the cholesteatoma is already far advanced. The cholesteatoma is usually diagnosed by a physician examining the ear with an oto-scope for routine surveillance. A shiny white collection of debris in the upper portion of the eardrum is a typical appearance.

The size of the cholesteatoma cannot be estimated from the visible portion. What looks like a small cholesteatoma may be the visible portion of an extensive cholesteatoma that has already invaded the bones of the skull. The cholesteatoma may or may not be associated with a foul smell coming from the ear.

## ➤ How is a cholesteatoma treated?

The treatment of a cholesteatoma always involves surgery. The earlier a cholesteatoma is caught, the more effective the surgery at restoring the child to health. Unfortunately, if the tiny bones of the middle ear, or the auditory nerve, or other sensitive struc-tures have been eaten through, they will not grow back.

It is far more effective to prevent cholesteatoma formation. This can be done by effective treatment of ear infections, along with continued observation of children who are otitis prone. If a retraction pocket becomes visible on physical examination, it should be promptly treated by the placement of ear tubes.

## ➤ *What is mastoiditis?*

The mastoid process, immediately behind the ear, begins life as mostly solid bone. Early on, a labyrinth of interconnecting air cells begins to form in the bone. This process is complete when a child reaches five to 10 years of age. These air cells connect to the middle air space.

These air cells are lined with a soft, glistening skin similar to that which lines the middle air space. When a child develops AOM, the lining of the mastoid air cells also becomes inflamed. Typically, as AOM resolves, the inflammation in the mastoid air space also resolves. Sometimes, however, infection is trapped in the mastoid process. When this happens, an abscess (a collection of infected pus) forms. This abscess grows and begins to erode the thin, bony walls.

Then the pus may spread in any of several directions. If it breaks through into the middle ear space, the mastoiditis is generally not very serious. The pus can, however, burrow under the skin or through other bones of the skull to cause very serious infections.

Before antibiotics were commonly used to treat ear infections, mastoiditis was a common complication of AOM and a frequent cause of death. A 90 percent reduction in the mortality rate occurred during the first decade that antibiotics were used to treat ear infections. In locations where antibiotics are not commonly available or where they are intentionally not used, the rate of mastoiditis is high.

## ➤ *How is mastoiditis diagnosed and treated?*

Children with mastoiditis generally have both a fever and inflammation (swelling, redness, and tenderness) of the ear or the skin behind the ear. Often the ear is prominently sticking out from the head, pushed forward by swelling of the mastoid process.

Mastoiditis should be suspected in any case of chronic purulent otitis media. Children with mastoiditis should receive aggressive treatment. This generally includes both intravenous antibiotics and surgery.

## ➤ *What is ossicular discontinuity?*

The ossicles are the tiny chain of bones that conduct sound across the middle ear space from the eardrum to the oval window of the cochlea. This chain of bones can be disconnected by retraction pockets, cholesteatomas, or even a simple perforation of the eardrum. Sometimes the ossicles are actually destroyed by mastoiditis or a cholesteatoma. As one might expect, **ossicular discontinuity** can cause the maximum conductive hearing loss possible—up to 60 decibels, making one unable to hear normal speech.

Ossicular discontinuity can often be detected upon simple physical examination of the ear with an otoscope. Hearing tests, otomicroscopes, and CAT scans can also aid in the diagnosis. Ossicular discontinuity requires surgical correction.

## ➤ *What is labyrinthitis?*

Sometimes an infection in the middle ear space spreads into the cochlea across the round window. The cochlea is the essential organ of hearing, where sound waves are transformed into nerve signals. In addition, it is largely responsible for our ability to balance. The cochlea is sometimes called the labyrinth. An infection of the inner ear is called **labyrinthitis**.

The main symptoms of labyrinthitis are sensorineural hearing loss and vertigo. Acute purulent labyrinthitis (an inner ear filled with pus) has become much less common since the advent of antibiotic therapy for AOM. Serous labyrinthitis (an inner ear filled with thin, clear fluid) is still relatively common.

Any child who has a history of AOM and sensorineural

hearing loss or vertigo should be carefully evaluated for the possible presence of labyrinthitis. Early treatment can help to preserve hearing.

Chronic labyrinthitis is usually the result of a cholesteatoma. The symptoms of chronic labyrinthitis are also hearing loss and vertigo, but they are of a subtle and insidious nature. Failure to diagnose cholesteatoma with chronic labyrinthitis can result in complete loss of hearing in the affected ear.

## Can an ear infection cause facial paralysis?

We get such delight from watching the facial expressions of our children. What a tragedy when these muscles are paralyzed by pressure on the facial nerve. Facial paralysis is not all that common, but at the major ear centers, such as the Children's Hospital of Pittsburgh, about one or two cases are seen every year. Initial treatment consists of ear tube insertion, drainage of the infection from the middle ear, and the administration of antibiotics. Usually, the paralysis improves rapidly. If it does not, or if other complications—such as mastoiditis or cholesteatoma—are found, then further surgery is immediately indicated.

## Does the eardrum become scarred after frequent ear infections?

The eardrum does not usually form true scars. But after frequent ear infections, whitish plaques often appear. These plaques contain calcium and phosphate crystals, left over from the body's attempts to heal the infections. This is called tympanosclerosis, or hardening of the eardrum.

Some children are genetically predisposed to tympanosclerosis. If these children have recurrent otitis media, the white plaques will form. The plaques are most common at the site of a healed hole in the eardrum, whether from spontaneous perforation or from ear tube placement.

As long as the white plaques are confined to the eardrum itself, there is little or no problem. Occasionally, the calcium and phosphate crystals trap the ossicles. If these tiny bones become trapped in the whitish plaques, then the child will have some degree of conductive hearing loss. This is quite rare, but if it occurs, it can be corrected with surgery.

## What is the significance of a blue eardrum?

A blue eardrum can be the hallmark of another complication of chronic otitis media called a **cholesterol granuloma**. This chronic collection of infection-fighting cells becomes a solid mass that cannot drain through the eustachian tube and cannot be drained by the insertion of ear tubes. Instead, a cholesterol granuloma can only be removed by more aggressive surgery.

## What do I do if the skin of the ear becomes red and crusty?

Sometimes an ear infection—particularly one in which the eardrum has been perforated—can spread into the skin of the external canal or even onto the skin of the outer ear. In this case, the skin becomes inflamed and usually forms a yellow, crusty layer on top. This condition is called **external eczematoid otitis**. The diagnosis should be confirmed by your physician since other conditions (such as **impetigo, seborrheic dermatitis**, and acute, diffuse external otitis) can look quite similar.

External eczematoid otitis can usually be effectively treated with a topical preparation that combines hydrocortisone and an antibiotic.

## Can an ear infection cause meningitis?

Bacteria infecting the middle ear can travel to the **meninges** (the protective tissue around the brain and spinal cord) in two different ways. Since the ear is so close to the brain and is connected to it by the auditory nerve, aggressive bacteria can directly invade to cause meningitis. In addition, bacteria from the ear can enter the bloodstream and travel within blood vessels to the meninges and cause meningitis.

Before the widespread treatment of ear infections with antibiotics, meningitis occurred in as many as one of every 50 children with ear infections. Thankfully, today this has become a rare problem in those parts of the world where antibiotics are used to treat ear infections. Still, for more than 20 percent of children who develop meningitis, ear infections are the apparent source.

## ➤ *Can an ear infection cause a brain abscess?*

An infection that begins in the ear and spreads can cause an abscess either within the brain itself or inside the skull, outside the brain. If the pus is trapped, it is called an abscess. If it is free flowing in the space between the brain and the skull, it is called **empyema.**

These complications, while once common, have become rare since the introduction of antibiotics. Nevertheless, when present, they still have a very high mortality rate—as high as 30 to 40 percent. More than half of those children who do recover are left with a permanent neurological deficit.

Children with this type of complication are very sick and are generally brought to medical attention quickly.

# 11

# Prevention

## How do I prevent swimmer's ear?

There are a couple of ways to prevent swimmer's ear. One is to make sure that your child's ears are completely dry after he has been in the water. This can be facilitated by having him tilt his head to one side and gently pull his ear in different directions to help the water to drain. It is also very helpful to carefully dry the opening of the ear, going as far in the ear as you can with a towel.

If swimmer's ear becomes a recurrent problem, you can put a few drops of rubbing alcohol in your child's ear each time it becomes wet to facilitate drying. An even better alternative is a few drops of a solution of one-third white vinegar and two-thirds rubbing alcohol. The acetic acid in the vinegar inhibits the growth of bacteria on the skin.

In most cases, earplugs do not help to prevent swimmer's ear. When an adhesive bandage is worn for a long time, the skin underneath becomes pale and waterlogged. Earplugs often produce a similar effect in the ear canal.

## How can I stop my child from getting otitis media?

It is far better to prevent an ear infection than to have to treat one after it has taken hold. Efforts at prevention involve avoiding exposure to ear infection-causing bacteria, increasing your child's immunity to the ear infection-causing bacteria, and ensuring proper functioning of the eustachian tube. Even with efforts in each of these three areas, some children will get ear infections. By taking these steps, however, the number of ear infections can be significantly decreased, and the duration and severity of these ear infections can likewise be ameliorated.

## How do I help my child to avoid the germs associated with ear infections?

This portion of prevention is easy to understand, but unfortunately, it's often very difficult to implement. As I described in chapter 4, the steady increase in ear infections among children parallels the steady increase in day-care centers. By minimizing the number of children to which your child is exposed, particularly during the winter months, you can decrease his risk of ear infections.

Keep in mind that most otitis-prone children have most of their ear infections in the 18-month window between six and 24 months of age. Of those 18 months, only a few will occur in late fall or winter. Thus, a decision to change your child's day-care arrangement is not necessarily a long-term proposition. A group size of six or fewer children results in measurably fewer infections (*Pediatric Clinics of North America,* December 1996). By moving your child to a smaller day-care setting during these months, you may actually save money. Look for a situation with minimal turnover of providers and children.

Hiring a nanny may be even better. If this isn't practical, you might consider sharing a nanny with another family. This option usually costs about the same as a group day-care setting and results in dramatically fewer exposures.

### ➤ *How else can I help my child to avoid ear infection-causing germs?*

The respiratory infections that lead to ear infections are often transmitted by touch or by fomites (pacifiers, toys, and other objects that carry germs). Frequent hand washing (especially before your child eats) and frequent washing of toys (particularly after they have been played with by someone else) are both helpful.

Respiratory infections can also be passed through the air. Try to avoid staying in small rooms with many sick people and poor circulation—such as movie theaters and airplanes, particularly in the winter—for long periods of time. Fresh air and air filters (especially HEPA filters) decrease the concentration of germs in the air.

Finally, avoid the overuse of antibiotics. Children who are frequently treated with antibiotics for viral infections or minor respiratory infections are the very children who have colonies of resistant, ear infection-causing bacteria thriving in their own noses and throats.

### ➤ *How do I boost my child's immunity against the organisms that cause ear infections?*

Breast-feeding gives your child a great start in developing his own immunity. The highest incidence of ear infections occurs between six and 12 months of age. If your child is otitis prone (especially if your child has ear infections before six months of age or you have another child who is otitis prone), breast-feeding throughout the first year can be particularly helpful. Even a few weeks of breast-feeding, however, results in fewer infections throughout the first three years of life.

## ➤ *Are there any vaccines against the bacteria that cause ear infections?*

The bacteria that most commonly cause ear infections (and sinus infections, for that matter) are *Streptococcus pneumonaie,* or pneumococcus. Current vaccines effectively immunize against the 23 subspecies of *Strep pneumo.* This does not prevent infections by other bacteria, but it does prevent infections by the bacteria that are the most difficult to treat after the fact.

The vaccine is very well tolerated by children. Most have minimal pain and redness at the site of the injection, and a few develop fevers. No serious reactions have been reported in children. Protection begins about two weeks following the injection. The vaccine is quite effective in children after their second birthdays, particularly when used in conjunction with prophylactic antibiotics. As the prevalence of antibiotic-resistant *Strep pneumo* increases, the importance of the pneumococcal vaccine increases as well.

The pneumococcal vaccine has been used to prevent ear infections in some children since 1975. The vaccine can be given before the second birthday, but it doesn't do much to build immunity against *Strep pneumo* at that time. Still, a child who receives the pneumococcal vaccine early can get a booster dose after his second birthday and not lose any of the potency of the vaccine. A newer, conjugate version of the vaccine has been developed that can be effective in children as young as three months. Trials are currently under way in several centers to determine the best use of this vaccine.

## ➤ *Is there a vaccine against* Haemophilus influenzae?

The *H. flu* vaccine, or Hib (for *Haemophilus influenzae* type b), has become a standard part of childhood immunization. Since the vaccine's introduction, serious *H. flu* disease, such as meningitis, has declined sharply.

The species of *H. flu* that cause ear infections are not type b. In fact, they are nontypeable *H. flu* since they lack the proteins on their coats with which typing is done. For this same reason, attempts to develop a vaccine against nontypeable *H. flu* using traditional vaccine development techniques have met with failure. Recently, scientists at St. Louis University have had some success in making a vaccine for the high-molecular-weight proteins that are used by the bacteria to adhere to tissues. This has resulted in a 50 percent decrease in *H. flu* ear infections in tested chinchillas. These high-molecular-weight proteins may be an important part of a new multicomponent vaccine. Work is actively under way toward a vaccine for humans (*Journal of Pediatrics,* February 1995).

## Is there a vaccine against Moraxella catarrhalis?

A paper from Helsinki University Hospital in Finland, published in the June 1995 issue of the *International Journal of Pediatric Otorhinolaryngology,* reports progress in the work toward an *M. cat* vaccine. The researchers suggest the very real possibility of an ear infection vaccine that would stimulate antibodies to *Strep pneumo, H. flu,* and *M. cat* and presumably significantly reduce the rate of infection, at least by the bacteria that have developed resistance to our antibiotics. This, coupled with wiser antibiotic practices, could greatly improve the situation in the future.

## Are there any other promising new vaccines?

Respiratory syncytial virus (RSV) commonly causes respiratory infections in children. These children produce large amounts of mucus. Recently, immunization against RSV has become possible. A study from Children's Hospital, Denver, published in the *Journal of Pediatrics* (August 1996), looked at the rate of ear infections in children who received RSV **immune globulin**. Some of the children received immunization, while some received a placebo. Researchers examined the children's ears without knowing who had been immunized. After the results were tallied, it was discovered that nonimmunized children had five times as many ear infections as their immunized counterparts.

Currently, the only version of RSV protection that is available must be given intravenously, is effective for only one month, and costs $1,000 per dose. While these considerations make the vaccine impractical for general use, the results of the study are very encouraging about what stands to be accomplished as better immunization becomes available. Even dropping the number of ear infections by 5 percent would have a big impact on our health and our economy. Dropping the number by 80 percent, which might soon be possible, would save billions of dollars and add greatly to the health of our children.

## What do I need to know about immune globulin?

For more than 35 years, some investigators have been suggesting that giving immune globulin (also called **gamma globulin** or immunoglobulin) to children would help to prevent ear infections. A blood test can be given to determine if a particular child has a low level of immune globulin. For children who continue to have frequent ear infections after the pneumococcal vaccine, antibiotic prophylaxis, and other preventive measures have been administered, testing total immune globulin levels may identify those who would get fewer episodes of otitis media while receiving immune globulin. When a child's total immune globulin levels are tested, it's also a good idea to test for the individual subtypes. A child may have a deficiency of one of the subtypes and still have a normal total amount. Even if a deficiency is detected, when immune globulin is given as a medicine, it is a human blood product that is given. It is made from the pooled blood plasma of many donors. Although it is now regarded as safe, it has been known to transmit the hepatitis virus. Use of immune globulin (or any therapy, for that matter) makes sense only when the benefits outweigh the risks.

### Does stress affect immunity?

Good nutrition (particularly adequate protein, vitamin, and mineral intakes), plenty of sleep, and decreased stress all help to bolster the immune system.

Ensuring good nutrition is probably the easiest of these three, but toddlers and two-year-olds can be quite picky eaters. If this is the case, you might enjoy Ellyn Satter's book *How to Get Your Kid to Eat...But Not Too Much* (Bull Publishing, 1987). You may also want to give a multivitamin as a safety net for those days when your child doesn't otherwise take in adequate nutrients.

Changing the stressors and the sleep patterns of your child can be quite difficult. While doing so should help to reduce the frequency of ear infections, the effect has not been measurable. I wouldn't lose too much sleep over these issues. But if you have an otitis-prone child, these issues might come into play in one very important decision: when to have another child.

Consider ear infections when deciding on the timing of another child. A new sibling is a source of stress and a reservoir for germs. You may want your second child to come along after your first child has begun to have fewer ear infections.

The question of stress may also come into play when you're

contemplating a move. Consider whether, on balance, the new living situation would be likely to increase or decrease the number of ear infections.

## ➤ How can I aid proper working of the eustachian tube?

The single greatest risk factor in eustachian tube dysfunction is cigarette smoke exposure. If your child is otitis prone, take whatever steps possible to keep him away from cigarette smoke. If possible, do not permit smoking in your home. If cigarette smoke can be smelled in the home, then a HEPA filter, fresh air, houseplants, and a fresh coat of paint can help to decrease your child's exposure level.

## ➤ Does position affect the eustachian tube?

The eustachian tube drains most effectively when the child is in an upright position. An angle of even 20 degrees above the horizontal offers a measurable advantage over lying flat. This is particularly important during feeding. Having your child eat and drink in as upright a position as practical will prevent some ear infections.

## ➤ Do allergies affect eustachian tube function?

The role of allergies in blocking the eustachian tube is an area of active investigation. Since allergies are difficult to reliably diagnose or exclude in very young children, clarification of this relationship remains difficult. Currently, though, it's estimated that 35 to 40 percent of ear infections have an allergic component. Swelling and blockage of the eustachian tube is the most studied mechanism, but substances that the body releases as part of the allergic response (such as eosinophil cationic protein and myeloperoxidase) are being found in middle ear effusions.

Otitis-prone children who have histories of eczema and/or

wheezing, who have many allergies in the family, or who have hay fever symptoms may greatly benefit from allergy control. Depending on the age of the child, some idea of what he is allergic to may be obtained through blood or skin tests.

Dust is the most common airborne allergen. Dust-proofing your child's room, while difficult, may have a large impact (see below). Mold spores are the second most common airborne allergen. Again, environmental control is the best way to go. Pets are another possible allergen source and should especially be kept from the room in which your child is sleeping.

Some studies suggest that allergies to foods, particularly dairy products, are more common in children who are otitis prone. Eliminating dairy products from the diet may be difficult but may be worthwhile for otitis-prone children with allergic histories.

Use of a topical nasal steroid (such as Beconase, Flonase, Nasacort, or Vancenase) or inhaled cromolyn (such as Nasalcrom) can reduce swelling in and around the eustachian tube in children with allergies. Again, antihistamines and decongestants have not been shown to help.

### How do I keep house dust away from my child?

This is no easy task! Dust control measures begin with eliminating the places where dust is most likely to collect. The child's room should have wood or linoleum flooring and no rugs of any kind. Toys should be wood, plastic, or metal—no stuffed animals or fabric toys. Venetian blinds are another dust collector to be avoided. Simple furniture collects less dust. Picture frames and pennants are both dust catchers.

Dust control is especially important where your child sleeps. The mattress should be encased in an allergen-proof zippered cover (such as Gore-Tex), and the zipper should be taped over. Use washable cotton or synthetic blankets, not fuzzy ones. The pillow should be Dacron or another synthetic fiber—no kapok, down, feathers, or foam rubber. The pillow also needs to be in a sealed case. Keep the bed as far as possible from an air vent.

Dust control also means relentless cleaning. As a start, wet-dust the room at least daily.

As you can see, this is a major task. It's probably best undertaken after a blood test or skin test has confirmed that your child has a dust allergy.

## How do I reduce mold in my home?

Unfortunately, this can also be very difficult. Again, confirm a mold allergy before attempting these measures. Mold grows wherever moisture is likely to collect. Bathrooms are a favorite spot for mold. Frequently wash grout between the tiles. Clean behind the toilet, under the sink, and in the corners.

Don't allow clothing to remain damp. Dry it immediately after laundering. Vent the clothes dryer to the outside air. Find a spot for damp shoes to air out.

Discard stored foods at the very first sign of spoilage. Use a disinfectant spray on any dehumidifier, vaporizer, humidifier, or air conditioner. Paint any moist walls with a mold-inhibiting paint. Replace vinyl squares on floors with sheet vinyl. Avoid houseplants and dried flowers. Clear vegetation away from the area immediately surrounding the house.

Mold reduction can be worth the effort for the child who is truly allergic to mold. The final suggestions require much less effort.

## Does getting a flu shot help?

This bit of preventive medicine is simple, quick, and discrete. Does it work? A study published in the *American Journal of Diseases of Children* (April 1991) demonstrated a 36 percent reduction in the rate of otitis media during flu season in those children who got flu shots, compared with those who didn't. By avoiding the flu, these children presumably kept their eustachian tubes unblocked and the drainage mechanism in better working order.

### ➤ *Is there an even simpler prevention idea?*

We know that in children, the eustachian tube drains optimally during swallowing, yawning, and crying. I recommend giving a younger child something to drink or having an older child chew sugarless gum or suck on sugarless candy during airplane descent, in order to facilitate opening of the tube at the critical time. Drinking plenty of water also helps to thin the nasal secretions and make blockage of the eustachian tube less likely.

I suggest that these same simple measures be used frequently throughout the day to improve eustachian tube function in otitis-prone children. They are safe, simple options that are consistent with the best available knowledge about ear infections. They could be especially useful during the first several hours that an infection is brewing and might help the body to fight it off without antibiotics.

### ➤ *Is any particular type of gum better than others?*

Recent evidence suggests that chewing gum that contains xylitol can prevent ear infections. The *xyl-* in xylitol comes from the Greek word *xylan,* meaning wood. Xylitol is a sugar made from wood.

Xylitol can be made from the cell walls of most land plants. Xylan, the naturally occurring substance that yields xylitol when refined, is most commonly found in straw, corncobs, oat hulls, cottonseed hulls, and wood. Xylitol is a common food sweetener. Unlike most sugars, which have six carbon atoms, this naturally sweet substance has only five.

While other sugars tend to promote the growth of bacteria, xylitol has been proven to inhibit the growth of bacteria. In particular, it has been shown to be effective in preventing dental cavities by inhibiting *Streptococcus mutans,* the main bacteria responsible for cavities.

Since the major cause of ear infections is *Streptococcus pneumoniae,* a species of bacteria closely related to *Strep mutans,* perhaps xylitol would prove effective in preventing ear infections. Researchers in Finland tested this hypothesis and published the results of their investigation in the November 9, 1996, *British Medical Journal.*

The study included 306 children in day-care nurseries, most of whom had histories of repeated ear infections. Half of the children chewed xylitol-sweetened gum (two pieces five times a day, after all meals and snacks); the other half chewed ordinary gum at the same frequency. During the two months of the study, 21 percent of the regular gum chewers and 12 percent of the xylitol gum chewers had one or more ear infections. Gum chewing itself probably prevented some ear infections by promoting swallowing and thus clearance of the middle ear. The sugar in the regular gum may have offset this effect by promoting bacterial growth in the children who chewed that gum. Still, in this study, xylitol dropped the incidence of ear infections by almost half!

Children in the xylitol group consumed a total of 8.4 grams of xylitol daily. Most had no side effects; two developed diarrhea, a known side effect of xylitol and other sweeteners.

A small number of children, almost all of them of Jewish descent, have a congenital enzyme defect that makes them unable to digest xylitol. This condition is called pentosuria. There are no associated disabilities. No treatment or dietary restriction is necessary. The xylitol is absorbed into the body and then excreted in the urine. The only problem arising from pentosuria is that children having this sugar in the urine sometimes are mistakenly diagnosed with diabetes and receive treatment for the condition. Pentosuria has no relationship to diabetes. Children with pentosuria could still use xylitol to prevent ear infections.

The Finnish study, which makes use of the natural, gentle antibiotic properties of plants, is an exciting development. While much research remains to be done, xylitol seems to be a safe and effective way to reduce the number of ear infections. I suspect it will also prove useful in preventing sinus infections since the same bacteria are involved.

# EPILOGUE

As you can tell by reading this book, there isn't one set of clear-cut answers when it comes to the treatment of ear infections. Physicians must consider what type of ear infection a child has and which bacteria are the culprits. The age of your child and the season of the year should both be considered, as should your child's response history and the resistant strains of bacteria in any given locality. Only after considering all of these factors can the doctor determine the best course of action. Even then, experimentation and observation are required to chart the best possible course for your child.

It is my hope that by being equipped with the information in this book, you will be able to form a partnership with your child's doctor in making decisions regarding your child's ear infection treatment. Along the way, if you have feedback or additional questions, please feel free to submit them to "Dr. Greene's HouseCalls" at http://www.drgreene.com.

Mention that you have read this book, so I will know how to better address your concerns. You can also log on to "HouseCalls" to get the most up-to-date information on ear infections and other pediatric issues. I hope you have enjoyed this book, and I hope to meet you on-line!

# GLOSSARY

**Abscess:** A localized collection of pus in a space formed by the destruction of surrounding tissue.

**Acoustic otoscope (or Reflectometer):** A handheld machine that uses sound waves to test for the presence of fluid in the middle ear. The machine looks much like an otoscope. It is sometimes used in the doctor's office to confirm or clarify what is found by direct visual examination of the eardrum with an otoscope.

**Acute otitis media (AOM):** An infection in the middle ear. Children with AOM have fluid in the middle ear accompanied by signs and symptoms such as ear pain, marked redness of the eardrum, and distinct distortion of the eardrum. Children with AOM act sick (especially at night) and often have fevers.

**Antibodies:** Any of a large number of protein molecules created in the body to recognize, combine with, and neutralize specific infectious agents or allergens. Antibodies are an important part of the immune system.

**Antihistamine/decongestant combinations:** Multisymptom cold medicines that contain both an antihistamine and a decongestant. An antihistamine is a compound that treats allergy and cold symptoms, including itching and swelling, by blocking part of the body's allergic response. A decongestant is a medicine that relieves the congestion of the mucous membrane by constricting the tiny blood vessels there.

**Anvil:** See **Incus**.

**AOM:** See **Acute otitis media**.

**Asthma:** A condition characterized by recurrent bouts of breathing difficulty, often with wheezing or coughing, that results from narrowing of the airways. Bouts of asthma can be provoked by a variety of factors, including allergies, irritants, exercise, and cold air.

**Audiometer:** An electronic device used for testing hearing. The instrument emits sounds of known frequency and intensity. The person being tested indicates when and where sounds are heard. For very young children, another device, which measures brain waves, can be used to tell if the child has heard the signal.

**Broad-spectrum antibiotics:** Drugs that are effective against a wide range of bacterial species.

**Capillaries:** Any of the tiny, thin-walled blood vessels throughout the body that carry blood between the smallest arteries and the smallest veins. Capillaries are less than one-fiftieth of an inch long and only as big around as a red blood cell.

**Cholesterol granuloma:** A chronic collection of cholesterol crystals and infection-fighting cells that have coalesced into a solid mass. A cholesterol granuloma is a serious complication of long-standing otitis media.

**Chorda tympani:** The nerve that originates from the facial nerve and, among other things, controls the tongue. It is often visible through the eardrum with an otoscope.

**Chronic purulent otitis media:** An ear infection that results in a perforation of the eardrum, which continues to drain pus over a long period of time. Chronic purulent otitis media is a serious infection that is much more difficult to treat than either acute otitis media or otitis media with effusion. It is often associated with other complications such as mastoiditis and cholesteatoma.

**Cilia:** Tiny vibrating hairs on the free surfaces of cells. On some cells, they beat rhythmically to propel mucus across the surface.

**Circadian rhythms:** The rhythmic repetition of certain bodily functions at about the same time each day. The word *circadian* comes from *circa,* meaning about, and *dies,* meaning day. The circadian rhythms affect things such as sleep and hormone levels.

**Cleft palate:** A split in the roof of the mouth that occurs as a birth defect.

**Cochlea:** The spiral structure in the inner ear that transforms sound waves into nerve impulses, which are sent to the brain.

**Colitis:** Inflammation of the colon. Colitis can result from many disease processes but can also be a side effect of antibiotic use.

**Conductive hearing loss:** Hearing loss that results from the failure of sound waves to reach the cochlea. This could be due to blockage of the ear canal, damage to the eardrum, fluid in the middle ear, ossicular discontinuity, and so on.

**Cortisol:** An important steroid hormone manufactured in the adrenal gland and secreted in a circadian rhythm. This life-maintaining hormone is especially important during periods of stress. Cortisol is also called hydrocortisone, particularly when it is manufactured synthetically.

**Culture:** The process of growing bacteria or other living material in a nutrient-rich environment that is especially conducive to its growth. In a diagnostic culture, a specimen (of blood, urine, mucus, or some other bodily fluid) is taken from the body and incubated to see what bacteria will grow.

**Down syndrome:** A congenital condition caused by an extra copy of chromosome 21. Children with Down syndrome often have mental retardation, slanting eyes, and a broad, short skull. Down syndrome is named after nineteenth-century English physician John Langdon Haydon Down, who first described the condition.

**Ear canal:** The passage leading from the external ear opening to the eardrum. This gently curved, skin-lined tube that travels through the bones of the skull goes by many names. In medical articles, you might also see it called the external auditory canal, the external acoustic meatus, or the *meatus acusticus externus*.

**Eardrum:** See **Tympanic membrane**.

**Ear tubes (or PE tubes, Grommets, Tympanostomy tubes, or Tympanotomy tubes):** Small, double-flanged tubes that are surgically inserted through the eardrums to prevent middle ear infections and to allow drainage when infections do occur. These tubes are made from a variety of materials, including metals and plastics. They are intended to function as an alternative to the eustachian tube when the eustachian tube is blocked.

**Eczema:** A condition of the skin characterized by red, itchy, scaly patches. This can be a chronic condition and is often associated with allergies and/or asthma. Patches of eczema can occur almost anywhere on the skin but most often appear in the flexes of the knees and elbows.

**Empyema:** The accumulation of a large amount of pus in a cavity of the body. This is the result of a serious infection.

**ENT:** An ear, nose, and throat specialist, sometimes called an otolaryngologist or otorhinolaryngologist.

**Eustachian tube:** The drainage tube that connects the middle ear to the back of the throat. The end of the tube closest to the ear is bony walled; the other end is made from cartilage. The entire length is lined by a mucous membrane. In the medical literature, it is also called the *tuba acustica* or *tuba auditiva*. (By the way, sixteenth-century Italian anatomist Bartolomeo Eustachio first discovered this structure. New generations of bacteria discover it every day.)

**External eczematoid otitis:** A yellow, crusted inflammation of the skin of the external ear canal or the external ear that results from otitis media spreading through a perforated eardrum. This is not a serious complication.

**False-positive:** A test result that wrongly indicates that a person has the condition for which he was tested.

**Fluorescence emission spectrophotometry:** The science of identifying substances based on the unique spectrum of light they emit. Fluorescent substances are those that emit light when struck by light. A fluorescence emission spectrophotometer functions by shining light at something and then recording the spectrum of light that shines back at the machine. Different substances have different "signature" or "fingerprint" patterns of light that they fluoresce. This type of technology holds great promise for identifying specific bacteria without the need for obtaining samples for culture.

**Fomite:** An object that retains bacteria when touched by a contagious person. The fomite may then spread the infection to someone else. Common fomites include cups, toys, books, and facial tissues.

**Gamma globulin:** See **Immunoglobulin**.

**Glue ear:** Otitis media accompanied by a thick, stubborn effusion. "Glue ear" is sometimes used interchangeably with "chronic otitis media with effusion" since it was once thought that the effusion always got thicker as time progressed.

**Grommets:** See **Ear tubes**.

**Group A *Streptococcus*:** A type of bacteria that causes infections in humans. Under a microscope, these bacteria look like a string of pearls. They are capable of bursting red blood cells. These bacteria are responsible for strep throat. They can also cause infections in other parts of the body, including, on occasion, the ear.

***Haemophilus influenzae* (or *H. flu*):** A type of bacteria that causes infections in humans. Under a microscope, they appear as tiny purple rods. They need fresh blood to meet their nutritional needs. *Haemophilus influenzae* type b (Hib) causes very serious infections, including meningitis. Nontypable *Haemophilus influenzae* is not as aggressive but is one of three types of bacteria that most commonly cause ear and sinus infections.

**Hammer:** See **Malleus**.

***H. flu*:** See *Haemophilus influenzae*.

**Immune globulin:** See **Immunoglobulin**.

**Immunoglobulin** (or **Gamma globulin** or **Immune globulin**): A protein of animal origin with known antibody activity.

**Immunologic:** Pertaining to the body's complex self-defense system against bacteria, viruses, yeast, and harmful cells.

**Impetigo:** A superficial infection of the skin, usually caused by streptococcal or staphylococcal bacteria.

**Incus (or Anvil):** The middle of the three tiny bones of the middle ear that conduct sound from the eardrum to the inner ear.

**Labyrinthitis:** An infection of the inner ear. Sometimes the infection in the middle ear space spreads into the cochlea across the round window. The cochlea is the essential organ of hearing, where sound waves are transformed into nerve signals. In addition, it is largely responsible for the ability to balance. The cochlea is sometimes called the labyrinth.

**Maintenance antibiotic:** See **Prophylactic antibiotic**.

**Malignant otitis externa:** Rapidly spreading otitis externa, especially when seen in someone with diabetes or an immune deficiency. Unlike most instances of otitis externa, this is a serious infection. It should be treated promptly and aggressively.

**Malleus (or Hammer):** The largest of the three tiny bones of the middle ear. It attaches to the eardrum. The clublike head of the malleus attaches to the incus (anvil).

**Mastoiditis:** An infection of the mastoid process. This aggressive, destructive infection can be a serious complication of an ear infection.

**Mastoid process:** A round knob of bone that can be felt just behind the lower edge of the ear. *Mastoid* means breast-shaped. This bone contains a labyrinth of tiny, thin-walled cells that connect to the middle ear.

*M. cat*: See *Moraxella catarrhalis*.

**Meninges:** The three membranes that surround the brain and the spinal cord. Inflammation of the meninges is called meningitis.

*Moraxella catarrhalis* (or *M. cat*): A type of bacteria that causes infections in warm-blooded animals, including humans. Under a microscope, they appear as short, unmoving, purple rods. They are one of three types of bacteria that most commonly cause ear infections and sinus infections.

**Mucous blanket:** The very thin, moving layer of mucus that rests on the cilia. This constantly moving blanket acts as a conveyer belt to move organisms and unwelcome particles out of the body. The mucous blanket is propelled by the cilia.

**Mucus:** A slippery, slimy substance that is secreted by the lining of the ears, nose, throat, and breathing tubes. It functions to lubricate and protect the underlying structures.

*Mycoplasma*: The smallest known free-living organisms. These tiny organisms differ from bacteria in that species of *Mycoplasma* lack a cell wall and are surrounded by a characteristic membrane. *Mycoplasma* are an infrequent cause of ear infections. Studies that look at causes based on cultures of middle ear contents rarely find *Mycoplasma* since they can be difficult to culture. *Mycoplasma* should be suspected when there are blisters on the eardrum or when there is a concurrent respiratory infection in the chest.

**Nasal swab:** A sample taken from the nose by using a cotton-tipped stick. This sample is then cultured to test for the presence and identity of bacteria.

**Needle aspiration:** See **Tympanocentesis**.

**OME:** See **Otitis media with effusion**.

**Ossicle:** Any tiny bone. The term is most often used to refer to any of the three tiny bones of the middle ear.

**Ossicular discontinuity:** Disconnection of the tiny chain of bones that conducts sound across the middle ear space from the eardrum to the oval window of the cochlea. This chain of bones can be disconnected by retraction pockets, cholesteatomas, or even a simple perforation of the eardrum. Sometimes the ossicles are actually destroyed by mastoiditis or a cholesteatoma. This causes significant hearing loss.

**Otitis externa** (or **Swimmer's ear**)**:** An inflammation or infection of the skin lining the external ear canal. Bacteria normally live on the surface of this skin with no ill effect. If there is a break in the skin's normal barrier, however, the bacteria can get inside the skin and cause otitis externa.

**Otitis media:** Inflammation or infection of the middle ear. Otitis media is divided into two main types: acute otitis media and otitis media with effusion. While "ear infection" is a broad term that might encompass infections of the inner, middle, and outer ears, it is usually used to indicate otitis media. Otitis media implies the presence of fluid in the middle ear. It remains the most common diagnosis in both doctors' offices and emergency rooms.

**Otitis media with effusion** (or **OME, Secretory otitis media, Serous otitis media,** or **Silent otitis media**)**:** Fluid in the middle ear space without other symptoms. This fluid generally contains disease-causing bacteria. Nevertheless, antibiotics are often not required for treatment. Children with OME act as if they feel well. Pediatricians often discover OME during well-child examinations.

**Otomicroscope:** A precision microscope developed to improve the ability to see the small structures of the ear. This device provides both magnification and illumination. It is especially important for use during ear surgery.

**Otorrhea:** A discharge from the ear, especially of pus.

**Otoscope:** An instrument used for examining the inner ear.

**Oval window:** A thin membrane on the inner wall of the middle ear. It separates the middle ear from the cochlea of the inner ear. The stapes rests on the oval window. The chain of three bones receives sound waves from the eardrum and transmits and amplifies the sound through the oval window to the cochlea.

**Persistent acute otitis media:** Acute otitis media in which the symptoms clear but then recur while a person is still on antibiotics or within five days of finishing antibiotics.

**PE tubes:** See **Ear tubes.**

**Placebo:** An inert therapy used in a controlled experiment for comparison. For a preventive therapy to be proven effective, it must be more effective than a placebo.

**Pneumatic otoscopy:** The process of assessing eardrum mobility by squeezing a little rubber bulb attached to the side of an otoscope. When the otoscope is in the child's ear canal, the bulb is lightly squeezed while the examiner watches to see if the eardrum moves. Then the observer lets go of the bulb, applying negative pressure, and again watches to see if the eardrum moves.

**Pneumococcus:** See *Streptococcus pneumoniae.*

**Preventive antibiotic:** See **Prophylactic antibiotic.**

**Prophylactic antibiotic (or Maintenance antibiotic):** A medicine that is given to prevent ear infections. The idea behind prophylactic antibiotics is that by using a small dose of medicine over a prolonged period of time, one can decrease the amount of ear infection-causing bacteria living in the nose and throat. A child on maintenance antibiotics is still vulnerable to colds, pressure changes, and allergies that block the eustachian tube. But even if the tube is blocked, the rapid growth of bacteria necessary to produce an episode of acute otitis media is less likely to occur.

**Psychoneuroimmunology:** The study of the relationship between the mental or emotional state and the immune system. Stress has clearly been shown to weaken the activity of the immune system. The details of this interaction are still being worked out.

**Recurrent acute otitis media:** A bout of acute otitis media that occurs more than five days after a person finishes antibiotics for a previous bout and her symptoms have cleared.

**Reflectometer:** See **Acoustic otoscope**.

**Rhinoviruses:** Any of the group of viruses most known for causing the common cold. More than 100 distinct strains are known.

**Round window niche:** A round opening on the inner wall of the middle ear, covered by a thin membrane. This membrane vibrates with sound and helps to transmit sound waves to the cochlea.

**Seborrhea (or Seborrheic dermatitis):** A chronic inflammation of the skin, especially the scalp. Seborrhea is characterized by redness, scaling, and yellow, crusted patches. Usually, seborrhea itches.

**Seborrheic dermatitis:** See **Seborrhea**.

**Secretory otitis media:** See **Otitis media with effusion**.

**Sedimentation rate (or Sed rate):** A blood test that measures the rate at which red blood cells settle to the bottom of a tube of blood. The value is the number of minutes it takes for the cells to settle. An elevated value suggests the presence of inflammation or infection but does not pinpoint the location or cause.

**Sed rate:** See **Sedimentation rate**.

**Self-limited viral infection:** An infection from which a person may be expected to recover without any direct treatment.

**Sensitive:** A lab test that identifies most cases that are being looked for. While a sensitive test will not miss many people that should test positive, it may produce many false-positive results.

**Sensorineural hearing loss:** Hearing loss resulting from damage to the cochlea or acoustic nerve, the nerve that leads from the ear to the brain.

**Serous otitis media:** See **Otitis media with effusion**.

**Silent otitis media:** See **Otitis media with effusion**.

**Soft palate:** The soft, fleshy part of the roof of the mouth. The palate is the wall between the mouth and the inside of the nose. The hard palate is the bony front half of the palate, just behind the teeth. Farther back, the soft palate is composed of soft tissue without bone.

**Specific:** A lab test in which a positive result is very reliable but a negative result may or may not be reliable. A rapid strep test is a specific test. If it is positive, the person has strep. If it is negative, the person probably does not have strep—but might.

**Stapes (**or **Stirrup):** The innermost of the three tiny bones of the middle ear. It is shaped somewhat like a stirrup. Its base rests on the oval window.

*Staphylococcus aureus***:** A family of bacteria that commonly causes infections in humans. Under a microscope, they look like a cluster of grapes. They are an infrequent cause of ear infections. Staph infections usually result in a lot of pus.

**Steroid medications:** A large group of anti-inflammatory medicines. These are related to many of the hormones produced by the human body. Steroid medications have no clearly defined role in the treatment of ear infections. While steroids do help speed the resolution of otitis media with effusion, in most cases the risks exceed the benefits.

**Stirrup:** See **Stapes.**

*Strep pneumo***:** See *Streptococcus pneumoniae.*

*Streptococcus pneumoniae* (or **Pneumococcus** or *Strep pneumo***):** A type of bacteria that causes infections in humans. Under a microscope, these bacteria look like a string of pearls. They are the most common cause of ear infections. They are also the most common cause of lobar pneumonia and a frequent cause of meningitis. Resistant strains of *Strep pneumo* are becoming a significant problem.

**Swimmer's ear:** See **Otitis externa.**

**Tympanic membrane (**or **Eardrum):** The thin membrane separating the external ear canal from the middle ear. This membrane vibrates when exposed to sound waves. These vibrations are transmitted to the adjacent malleus.

**Tympanocentesis (**or **Needle aspiration):** The process of inserting a needle through the eardrum to remove fluid from the middle ear for evaluation or treatment. Needle aspiration is performed to culture the contents of the middle ear. The procedure may help to eliminate the infection.

**Tympanogram:** A graphic representation of the mobility of the eardrum obtained by tympanometry.

**Tympanometer:** An instrument used to assess the mobility of the eardrum by subjecting it to positive and negative pressures and recording the reflected sound waves.

**Tympanometry:** The process of assessing the mobility of the eardrum by subjecting it to various positive and negative pressures and recording the reflected sound waves.

**Tympanosclerosis:** Hardening of the eardrum. After frequent ear infections, whitish plaques often appear. These plaques contain calcium and phosphate crystals, which are left over from the body's attempts to heal the infections. The plaques are most common at the site of a healed hole in the eardrum. As long as the white plaques are confined to the eardrum itself, there is little or no problem. Occasionally, the calcium and phosphate crystals trap the ossicles. If these tiny bones become trapped in the whitish plaques, then a child will have some degree of conductive hearing loss. Otherwise, the hearing loss is negligible—less than 0.5 decibel.

**Tympanostomy tubes:** See **Ear tubes**.

**Tympanotomy tubes:** See **Ear tubes**.

**Vertigo:** A sensation that causes a person to feel as if the world were revolving around her or as if she were revolving in space.

**Viscosity:** The thickness of a fluid, or its resistance to flow.

# INDEX

## A

Abdominal pain, antibiotics and, 97

Abscesses
  brain, 171
  defined, 134, 189

Acetaminophen
  air travel and, 53
  effects, 73-74

Aconite, acute otitis media (AOM) and, 110

Acoustic otoscope, defined, 64, 189

Acute otitis media (AOM). *See also* Ear infections
  air travel and, 51
  antibiotics
    cure rate, 101-102
    effectiveness, 87, 101-102
    prophylactic, 124-125, 126
    treatment guidelines, 70-72
    treatment regimen, 74-75
  causes, 31
  complications, 102, 134
  defined, 26, 189
  delayed therapy, 71-72
  ear tubes and, 133-134, 135, 136-137

Inflammation, antibiotics
and, 72

Irritants, effects, 30, 55

# K

Keflex. *See* Cephalexin

Kidneys

amoxicillin and, 87

azithromycin and, 91

cefixime and, 93

trimethoprim-
sulfamethoxazole and,
100

# L

Labyrinthitis

defined, 168, 195

effects, 169

symptoms, 168-169

Language delay, defined,
158-159

Language development

ear infections and, 159-161,
163

stages, 158-159

Lemon juice with saline,
effects, 109-110

Lorabid. *See* Loracarbef

Loracarbef

administration with food,
84, 99

dosing schedule, 83, 86, 99

effects, 78, 86, 99

side effects, 99

storage, 83, 86, 99

taste, 81, 86, 99

# M

*M. cat. See Moraxella
catarrhalis (M. cat)*

Maintenance antibiotic,
defined, 87, 198-199

Malleus, defined, 22, 195

Mastoid process, defined,
23, 195

Mastoiditis

causes, 75

defined, 23, 167, 195

diagnosis/treatment,
167-168, 169, 195

eardrum perforation and,
162, 164

Measles-mumps-rubella
vaccine, ear infections
and, 52